Group Dynamics in Occupational Therapy

The Theoretical Basis and Practice Application of Group Treatment

Group Dynamics
in
Occupational Therapy

The Theoretical Basis
and Practice Application
of Group Treatment

Marilyn B. Cole, MS, OTR/L
Quinnipiac College
Hamden, Connecticut

PHILA. COLLEGE PHARMACY & SCIENCE
J. W. ENGLAND LIBRARY
4200 WOODLAND AVENUE
PHILADELPHIA, PA 19104-4491

RELEASED

SLACK Incorporated, 6900 Grove Road, Thorofare, NJ 08086-9447

Cover illustration originated by: Marilyn B. Cole, MS, OTR/L

Group dynamics in occupational therapy: the theoretical basis and practice application of group treatment/by Marilyn B. Cole.
  p. cm.
  Includes bibliographical references and index.
  ISBN 1-55642-119-2 (soft)
  1. Occupational therapy. 2. Group psychotherapy
  3. Small groups. I. Title.
  RC487.C65 1993
  616.89′165—dc20   93-27802

Published by: SLACK Incorporated
              6900 Grove Road
              Thorofare, NJ 08086-9447

Last digit is print number: 10 9 8 7 6 5 4 3 2

Contents

Contents

About The Author

Marilyn B. Cole, MS, OTR/L is an assistant professor of occupational therapy at Quinnipiac College, Hamden, Connecticut and an occupational therapy consultant. She holds a bachelor's degree in English from University of Connecticut, a graduate certificate in occupational therapy from University of Pennsylvania, and a master's degree in clinical psychology from University of Bridgeport. She is licensed by the state of Connecticut to practice occupational therapy, and is certified by the Center for Study of Sensory Integrative Dysfunction to administer the Southern California Sensory Integration Tests.

The author has over 24 years of clinical experience at Eastern Pennsylvania Psychiatric Institute, Middlesex Memorial Hospital, Lawrence and Memorial Hospitals as well as Newington Children's Hospital. She has also served as consultant for the West Haven V.A. Medical Center, the Portland Public Schools, Fairfield Hills Hospital and St. Joseph's Manor, all in Connecticut.

This is Marli Cole's eleventh year of full-time teaching. She has taught courses in psychiatric clinical media, group leadership, group dynamics, frames of reference, fieldwork I and II, psychopathology, sensory motor integration, geriatrics, computer technology lab and research.

Marli has published four professional journal articles and a chapter in *Group Process and Structure* (ed. Gibson 1988). She has presented papers and workshops at professional conferences on eighteen different topics. Marli has also delivered professional presentations to Yale psychiatric residents, the Connecticut Occupational Therapy Association, the American Occupational Therapy Association annual conferences in Philadelphia, Kansas City and New Orleans, and to the World Federation of OT annual congress in Melbourne, Australia.

Acknowledgments

For help with the revision of my group dynamics course that led me to write this book, I'd like to thank my colleagues and part-time instructors Rosanna Tufano, Sigita Banevicius and Betsey Smith, and my department chairperson, Muriel Lerner.

For painstaking review of my chapter drafts and for keeping me in touch with reality, I'd like to thank Valnere McLean, Mildred Ross, Barbara Neuhaus, Karen Macdonald, Ona Killough and Claudia Allen.

For the group protocol concept, I owe thanks to Anne Scott of SUNY Downstate Occupational Therapy Department in Brooklyn, who convinced me of its importance, and encouraged me to write this book.

For ongoing moral and emotional support and for keeping my writing on schedule (almost), I'd like to thank Anne Golenwsky, Amy Mims and Mary Rose Preston. For trying out the learning exercises presented in this text and for providing so many fine examples, I'd like to thank my occupational therapy students at Quinnipiac.

For help with word processing and encouraging smiles, I'd like to thank my daughter, Charlot.

Introduction

This book presents a unique point of view about occupational therapy group treatment: that all group treatment, whether we know it or not, is theory-based. Traditionally, group dynamics have been taught as a body of knowledge more or less separate from occupational therapy theory. Group dynamics are the forces that affect the interaction of group members to produce an outcome. The issues of group process, group development, leadership styles and group norms and roles were a focus of social psychology research in the mid-twentieth century. The outcomes of this early group research, including the work of Lewin, Bion, Tuckman, Benne and Sheats and many others, form the basis of what occupational therapy curriculums have defined as **group dynamics theory**.

Furthermore, the format for leading groups, such as that suggested by Howe and Schwartzberg, has traditionally been generic, that is, presented without an acknowledged bias toward any particular occupational therapy theory.

A theory defines the relationship between occurrences and explains why things happen. A theory is not a fact until it has been substantiated through research. A single theory can include many concepts or ideas. Occupational therapy uses many practice theories, or frames of reference. A frame of reference departs from pure theory when it applies the theory to a specific situation, such as patient treatment. The terms practice theory and frame of reference will both be used in this text to refer to this application to patient treatment.

The premise of this book is that neither group dynamics nor group format can be understood and used apart from theory. Both reflect a point of view which has a definite, although often unacknowledged, theoretical basis. All of the group techniques we know of patient treatment are influenced by the larger theoretical trends in our culture, such as in psychology, business management and medical research. This does not mean that we, the occupational therapy profession, have not developed our own theories. It simply means that we have not developed them in isolation. In this book, I have attempted to acknowledge the origins of many of the group techniques we have come to know as a part of occupational therapy.

My original concept in writing this text was to create a group dynamics workbook for my group dynamics classes. My need was to provide OT students a guidebook in the application of group dynamics theory and I wanted to make theory more concrete and usable in the clinic. Thus, this text begins by addressing the need for technique. Chapter 1, *Group Leadership*, suggests a concrete, seven step method of leading a group. This is a place to begin learning what OT group treatment is all about.

Likewise, in Chapter 2, *Understanding Group Dynamics*, the traditional body of knowledge about group dynamics is addressed in practical terms. The contributions of early research in social psychology and the writings on application of group psychotherapy by Irvin Yalom are acknowledged. However, these basic concepts are further developed and expanded in ways that are unique to occupational therapy group treatment.

Only when we reach Chapter 3 do we discover that both the seven step group technique and many of the principles of group dynamics have their roots in the existential/humanistic frame of reference. This context is not intended to limit our use of the techniques, but rather to expand it. The linking of the concepts of humanism and existentialism with an approach to group treatment is a good example of how occupational therapists can apply theory and use it as a guideline for treatment.

My approach to the seven frames of reference tends to be historical, and the concepts collected are often from the original authors/theorists. However, it should be emphasized that the chapters on practice theories (frames of reference) are not intended to be complete; rather, I have selected from these frames of reference those concepts that are most useful to us in planning and leading occupational therapy groups. I have attempted also to show how groups differ in each of the seven frames.

All of the chapters on group format, group dynamics and frames of reference (Chapters 3-9) will hopefully prepare the student for the final phase of occupational therapy group planning-writing a group protocol. The group protocol is a complete plan for group treatment, beginning with defining the population and ending with outlines of the specific group sessions to be included.

Guidelines for how to select a frame of reference and how to use *Uniform Terminology for Occupational Therapy* (1989) are a part of the group planning process outlined in Chapter 10. Chapter 11 offers an example of a group protocol, a group laboratory experience for students entitled *Developing Your Professional Self*. This series of group exercises serves three purposes. Besides giving an example of the protocol assignment, it suggests a professional growth experience for occupational therapy students and it gives students group experiences in which to observe and learn about group dynamics.

Hence, this text begins and ends with technique. Throughout the book are individual exercises intended to facilitate learning. The central portion on frames of reference represents an attempt to derive from theory what is useful when planning and leading occupational therapy groups. In this way, what I hope students will see is that applying theory is not a burden, but a way to guide our planning and make it easier. This book helps occupational therapy students to organize their thinking about our multiple practice theories and to apply them systematically to occupational therapy group treatment.

Bibliography

Howe M. and Schwartzberg S. *A Functional Approach to Group Work in Occupational Therapy*. Philadelphia: J.B. Lippincott, 1986.

SECTION ONE

Acquiring Group Skills

Introduction

This section begins with experiential learning. Chapter 1, *Group Leadership*, is basically in a "how to" format, which is intended as an introduction to therapeutic group leadership for beginning occupational therapy students. This is not to imply that the seven step format is the only way to lead groups, nor is it the best way for all patient groups. The basic premise of this text is, in fact, the opposite: that group leadership, structure, goals and activities all vary with each frame of reference as therapy groups are matched to different patient needs.

Chapter 2, *Understanding Group Dynamics*, selects from the vast body of knowledge about group dynamics, those elements of groups that have the most impact for occupational therapy. An understanding of the process of groups, group development, leadership styles, norms and roles, has a part in designing and leading activity groups. Guidelines on how to approach common member problems is also helpful to the beginning therapist. The learning activities suggested in Chapter 2 are intended to increase awareness of the more abstract aspects of group process. This is best accomplished when students personally go through a small group experience, such as the one described in Chapter 11, *A Group Laboratory Experience*. In this way, as students absorb the content of Chapter 2, they can apply the principles directly to their own experience.

Chapter

1

Group Leadership

It has been my observation during the last eleven years of teaching that students learn best by experience. They are anxious to know how to *do* occupational therapy. They are both eager and afraid to begin working with patients. To the beginning student, occupational therapy is just a label. Only when students are put in the role of a professional do they become aware of what needs to be learned.

Acting like a professional is often difficult for students, whose only experience in group leadership is usually with groups of their peers. Part of making the transition to a professional role is learning that it is different from a social role. Professionalism carries with it an authority and a directness of purpose which will need to be practiced by students before they begin interacting with patients.

This book begins with a technique which is a concrete form of group leadership training. This allows students to practice the role of a professional. It is as generic as any technique can be, and is intended as a beginning experience for students entering the profession. As the educational process continues, it is expected that the technique will be modified many times over to match the needs of each unique group. It is changed in content to meet new goals and address different age groups and disability areas. It is changed in process and structure to align with different frames of reference. But learning has to begin somewhere. Just as motor development precedes cognitive awareness in the infant, a concrete experience in group leadership becomes the forerunner of the knowledge and understanding of its purpose and application in treatment.

Seven Step Format for Activity Groups

These seven steps can meet the needs of the highest level groups, and so are very appropriate for student groups. They are chosen for maximum integration of learning by the members. It is clear that this format will not fit every need, goal or patient population. However, the format is easily adapted to meet the goals of any group. How and why it will be modified will be described later. The steps in group leadership are: 1) introduction, 2) activity, 3) sharing, 4) processing, 5) generalizing, 6) application and 7) summary. The original idea for this format comes from the Pfeiffer and Jones *Reference Guide to Handbooks and Annuals* (1977), which presents a five step format that is expanded and adapted for occupational therapy here.

Introduction

Let's assume the occupational therapist is leading the initial session of a group. The therapist does not know the members well, although it is presumed he or she knows who they are and something about their disability and the reasons they have been assigned to the group. (In many settings, the OT would select the members him/herself.) The members may not know one another. So once the group is gathered, the OT introduces him or herself to the group. This introduction includes the therapist's name, title and the name of the group that is about to begin. Then, even if people know one another, the therapist asks the members to greet the group by saying their names in turn. This procedure does more than just help the members learn one another's names, it acknowledges their membership in the group and invites them to be a part of it. In subsequent groups, it may not be necessary to say names around the room, but acknowledgment of each member's presence should still be done. A friendly "hello" or "welcome back" from the therapist may accomplish this.

Warm-up

The next thing the leader should be concerned with is the receptivity of the members. How alert are they? How preoccupied are they? How are they feeling? Are members ready to begin a new experience, or do they need to be "warmed up?" A **warm-up** is an exercise that captures the group's attention, relaxes them and prepares them for the experience to follow. Warm-ups can be structured or casual and impromptu. A nice collection of structured warm-up activities can be found in Rider and Gramblin's *Activity Card File* (1987). An example of a structured warm-up is "Grandma's Trunk." Each member says, "Grandma has an old trunk up in the attic and in it I found _____." Members fill in the blank by saying the name of something that begins with each letter of the alphabet in order. All items must be repeated each time. For example, the first person says she found an Acorn, the second found an Acorn and a Bonnet, etc. If there are eight members to the group, the eighth one must remember the seven items preceding his contribution.

This warm-up obviously requires members to have a good short-term memory. The occupational therapist should choose a warm-up that challenges members enough to hold their interest, but is not beyond their capabilities. Warm-up activities accomplish several important goals. The game creates an atmosphere of spontaneity and fun. It also refocuses members' thoughts from whatever they came to the group thinking about, to this group right here, right now. If a warm-up works properly, it gets the members listening for what will come next, and encourages their cooperation in the group experience to follow.

All groups do not need a formal warm-up. Sometimes the best warm-up is just a casual conversation about how members are feeling today. If the group is to engage in a discussion, just getting the members talking may prepare them adequately. If the agenda is more creative in nature, an imaginative warm-up may be in order. Remembering what happened last week may be an appropriate warm-up to an activity which will be the next step in a sequence. It is important to make the warm-up relevant to the activity to follow. One does not set a mood of fun and games when the agenda for the group is a serious issue like coping with loss, or finding new employment.

Setting the Mood

Setting an appropriate mood is an important objective in choosing the most appropriate warm-up. However, setting the mood for a group is not only accomplished with a warm-up. The environment, the therapist's facial expression and manner of speaking and the media used, all contribute to the mood. Care should be taken before the group begins, to set up the environment accordingly; this includes proper lighting, getting rid of clutter, setting out equipment, supplies and the correct number of chairs, and avoiding distractions as much as possible.

Expectation of the Group

The therapist's manner and expression should generally reflect his or her expectation of the group. A therapist cannot expect group members to take an activity seriously if the therapist does not appear to do so. The therapist will always be a role model to members, whether or not it is his or her intention. If the therapist begins by saying, "OK you guys, listen up!," the members will be expecting a pep talk before a football game, rather than a serious discussion about managing their time. A direct and authoritative presentation of the group is one of those skills students must learn that make up the role of the professional.

Explaining the Purpose Clearly

Clearly explaining the purpose of the group is a primary task in the introduction phase. How this is done depends on the type of group and the patients' level of understanding. This is a step that should *never* be left out. The intent of the group has undoubtedly been explained individually to each member why he/she was assigned to this particular group. But it should not be taken for granted that the patients remember, or even fully understand, the purpose of a group from a previous explanation. The purpose should be reiterated by the OT in a way the patients are likely to understand. A higher level group of patients will want to know why they are being asked to do a particular activity. If they are asked to do calisthenics, it will be helpful to tell them that physical exercise has been known to change brain chemistry, to relieve stress, to elevate their mood and to energize their muscles. Patients who understand and believe this will be much more willing to cooperate.

Lower cognitive level patients are unlikely to understand such abstract explanations of purpose. For them, a modified explanation such as, "these exercises will make you feel better so you can do more for yourself," may suffice. With severely ill patients, a friendly expression and a gentle touch that says, "trust me, this will help you" may enlist their cooperation.

We started out assuming that the OT is introducing a new group experience to a new set of patients. In an initial session, more time is taken in explaining the purpose than in subsequent sessions. In describing the purpose of the group, the goals of the whole series of group sessions should be outlined in the initial session. If possible, the goals should be spelled out in concrete terms. For example, money management is an activity of daily living that occupational therapists often help patients work on improving. In a money management group, members may be expected to plan and carry out a realistic budget for one month and keep accurate records in a notebook. Therapists often use behavior change as a measure of progress in their patients. When patients are informed about the behavior that is expected to change, they can keep track of their own progress. This becomes motivating when patients in groups start measuring each other's behavior change (or lack thereof). Peer pressure is a powerful motivator of change in human behavior.

Describing the purpose of each session will not take as much time as the initial explanation. However, the goals for each activity should always be stated clearly at the beginning of each session. Patients need to be reminded of how the group is expected to help them. As the therapist gets to know the members better, explanations can be more individualized and related to the problems each member presents. For example, in introducing a stress management session, the therapist might mention that: "In the previous sessions, you've been complaining about how difficult it is to carry out daily activities when you're feeling so much stress. Today's activity will give you some new strategies for reducing the stress in your lives." Generally, when patients are told exactly how an activity will help them, they are much more interested in doing it.

Brief Outline of the Session

Finally, the introduction ends with a brief outline of the session to immediately follow. The time frame, the media and the procedures are included. For example, if the activity for a one hour session is to "draw yourself," the therapist might say: "We will be using the paper and markers provided to do a drawing for the next 20 minutes. After we are finished, I will ask each of you to explain your drawing to the group and we will discuss the activity for the last half of the session." This explanation serves several purposes. It tells the patient how long he has to complete the activity. A complex artistic drawing cannot be done in 20 minutes, so if he is to finish, he knows he must keep it simple. The explanation also warns him that he probably shouldn't draw anything he doesn't wish to discuss. Although this may be seen as inhibiting the patient's creativity, it also allows him to control the image of himself he projects to the group. How the therapist handles this will depend on the goal of the activity. If self-awareness is more important than social awareness, the patients may be given the option *not* to explain everything about their drawing. They need only say as much as they are comfortable sharing.

As well as understanding the purpose of the drawing activity, patients will want to know what is to be done with it afterward. When they know they will be expected to talk about their work, their drawing may be more focused, and they will be more prepared to speak when it's their turn. It may be helpful to tell patients ahead of time whether their drawings will be kept by the therapist, or if they can keep them. The disposition of drawings produced will differ depending on the goals and the frame of reference used. However, stating the procedures ahead of time is most respectful to the patient and may also prevent difficulties later in the session.

The brief outline of the session also gives members a clue to the session's focus. The example given tells patients that the activity portion is relatively short (20 minutes) compared with the discussion portion (at least 30 minutes). Members will see that the focus is on the discussion rather than the drawing and on learning and interaction rather than artistic talent. The outline helps patients and therapist get the whole session in perspective.

The introduction is one of the steps that is consistently kept in every frame of reference and every type of group. The structure may become less formal, with practice, but the essential elements must remain. An introduction can make or break a group, and each element plays a part in the effectiveness of group outcome.

Activity

Many factors should be considered when planning the activity. In a professional setting, this is, in fact, a tremendously complex process. It incorporates all we know about patients; diseases; and their corresponding dysfunctions, assessment, treatment planning, activity analysis and synthesis and group dynamics. Selecting a therapeutic activity involves the entire process of clinical reasoning that occupational therapists take two or three years of academic training to learn. One of the problems in learning group technique before the theory, is that the process will seem oversimplified and incomplete. However, students should have a positive experience in trying out the role of an occupational therapist, even though there is much more to be learned before they can adequately do it in the clinic.

Designing the group experience is a very complex process and many issues should be considered. All of them cannot be addressed here. For the purposes of simplification, the following issues will be presented for consideration in selecting a therapeutic activity: timing, therapeutic goals, physical and mental capacities of the members, adaptation of an activity and knowledge of the therapist.

Timing

With five more steps to go, (sharing, processing, generalizing, application and summary), it should be evident that the activity to be experienced should be kept fairly simple and short. This will vary of course, but for our purposes in learning to plan and lead groups, the activity portion should last no longer than one third of the total session. For example, in this seven step process for a one hour group, the activity used must be adapted to fit a time frame of 15-20 minutes and to meet a preset therapeutic goal.

Goals

It is impossible to plan an activity without first planning and structuring the goals. Goals are desired outcomes, something patients and therapists strive together to accomplish. Setting therapeutic goals for patients involves assessing their needs and applying our knowledge of their abilities and disabilities. The referral source, such as the hospital treatment team, the doctor or the nursing home staff, may have already defined the problem, i.e., "this patient needs to develop adequate social skills," or " help patient to learn joint protection and energy conservation techniques." In planning our practice groups for peers, the student might first think about what goals might be useful for herself. Perhaps coping with stress, setting priorities, clarifying values, managing money, managing time and asserting oneself in social situations may be troublesome areas for students. The group goals should be chosen to meet the needs of most of the members.

Once the goal is defined, an activity is designed or selected to help members achieve that goal. For example, when goals have to do with personal growth, for example, creative activities such as drawing, sculpture, dramatics and storytelling can be helpful. Through the creative process, many parts of the self can be revealed and explored. If goals are more socially oriented, structured group tasks involving interaction of the members are appropriate, i.e., communication exercises or group decision-making and problem solving.

Physical and Mental Capacities of the Members

Selection of the activity or experience is further determined by the physical and mental capacities of the members. If members are college students around age 20, without physical or mental handicaps, the possibilities are almost unlimited. The challenge would be to find an activity that holds their interest and from which they can learn something new and meaningful. When members of the group are geriatric patients, the physical and fine motor components of the activity may be limited. A game of balloon volleyball or a lively discussion about a topic of interest might be suitable. When group members are mentally retarded, their cognitive limitations must be taken into account, and the activity will need to be more physical and concrete (not abstract) in nature. Cooking and simple crafts and games are often useful activities with the mentally retarded. Assessment of the physical and mental functioning of an individual is the subject of other textbooks in occupational therapy, and so will not be covered here. In the clinical setting, assessment would be done on each member prior to starting the group.

Knowledge and Skill of the Leader

A final factor in the activity selection process is the knowledge and skill of the leader. What activities are familiar to the leader that can be adapted to this group experience? Student leaders usually choose activities for the group that they, themselves are comfortable with or have done before. A student who has had dance lessons may feel very comfortable introducing a movement activity; a leader with artistic talent may choose a drawing activity. Crafts, games and educational or social experiences may be sources of familiar activities to be adapted. There are a wealth of resource books available offering ideas for structured experiences in human relations. An example is Rider and Gramblin's *Activity Card File* which is updated every few years. When using these references, it should be kept in mind that most of the exercises cannot be done as written, but will have to be adapted to the specific goals set by the occupational therapist.

Adaptation of an Activity

Adaptation of an activity requires some knowledge of activity analysis and synthesis. Activity analysis is the "process of examining an activity to distinguish its component parts. Activity synthesis is the process of combining component parts of the human and nonhuman environment so as to design an activity suitable for evaluation or intervention relative to . . . performance" (Mosey 1981, 114). The analysis of activities is the subject of other textbooks and will not be fully described here. This is yet another example of the complex process of clinical reasoning in occupational therapy, in bringing together concepts from many bodies of knowledge to influence our treatment choices.

Activity Analysis is the breaking down of an activity into its component parts and matching each part with the human functions required to accomplish it. Playing "Bingo", for example, may be analyzed as shown in Figure 1-1.

In this oversimplified illustration, the therapist must know 1) how to play Bingo and 2) what physical and mental skills are required to play. Knowing this, the patient's skill is matched with what is required to do the activity. Modifications can then be made in the activity to suit the patient's abilities. This is activity synthesis. For example, a group of patients with poor vision may need Bingo cards with larger letters and numbers and bright colored markers. A hearing impaired group will need to have the calls written on a blackboard or flashed on a screen. Patients with poor motor control may need a Bingo card with magnetic markers that will stay in place even if the card is moved. Higher functioning groups may need more challenging requirements to win, such as markers all

Playing Bingo	
Activity components	Skills needed
A letter and number are called	Patient must hear the call and associate it with written letters and numbers
The bingo card is scanned	Patient must read and understand written letters and numbers
A marker is placed on the number called	Patient must have eye-hand coordination, fine motor skills and grasp-release
When a row of five is marked	Patient must have good visual perception
Patient calls out "BINGO"	Patient must be able to speak loudly

Figure 1-1. Activity Analysis.

around the edge or in the shape of an "H" or an "S." Additional motivation may be built in by offering appealing prizes.

Once selected, the therapeutic activity should be presented in a systematic way. First, the activity should be explained as directly and simply as possible. Procedures and instructions are given in language appropriate to the level and background of the group. The therapist should get feedback from the group as to whether they understood the directions, and should answer any questions before proceeding. Materials and supplies, if needed, should be hidden from view until they are actually needed. As the activity is in progress, the therapist may choose to participate in order to avoid making members feel self-conscious or watched. However, a leader should not allow his or her participation to detract from making relevant observations of the group to be discussed later.

When the activity portion of the group is finished, any materials used such as pencils or paints, should be collected and placed out of sight before moving to the discussion stages. This will avoid having some members continue working after time is up, or be distracted by the extraneous items. It may be necessary to stop some individuals before they are finished in order to keep the group moving along. The leader needs to be prepared to continually adapt and structure the group.

Sharing

After completing the activity, each member is invited to share his own work or experience with the group. The structure and process for sharing may vary with each activity. If the activity involves drawing or writing something individually, members would show the drawing and explain it to the group, or read to the group what was written. In activities involving interaction, members share what the experience was like for them, or what it meant to them. In either case, the therapist is responsible for making sure each member has a chance to do this.

Another important responsibility in this phase is to make sure each member's contribution is acknowledged. Acknowledgment may be done verbally or non-verbally. Sometimes just a smile and a nod may be all that is necessary. Members often want to respond to one another's sharing, but the therapist may need to model this to be sure the responses show caring and concern. **Empathy** is an important factor here. This means the therapist responds to the patient in a way that communicates understanding of how the patient feels. Empathy will be discussed in more depth in a later chapter.

Some members may be reluctant to share, for various reasons. The therapist may need to support and encourage patients to share, or to reassure them that they can do it without negative consequence. However, if a patient refuses to share, this must be accepted; patients should not be unduly pressured to disclose anything about themselves that they don't feel comfortable sharing.

Generally, it doesn't matter in what order the members share, but often it is easier to keep track if members just go in order around the circle. It is usually best to ask for a volunteer to start the process, so that patients feel some control over the group. However, the therapist can start to role model for the group what is expected to be shared. For example, in the "Best Friend" exercise from Pfeiffer and Jones (1973), the therapist might begin by getting up and standing behind a chair and saying "This is my best friend Beth (indicating an invisible self in the empty chair). She's a person who likes cooking healthy food, doing creative projects and helping other people. Her pet peeve is people who smoke. She has always wanted to write a book...etc." The therapist models the format the members will use in sharing.

There are a few activities for which sharing is not a separate step, but is incorporated into a discussion activity. For example, "Moral Decisions" is a group decision-making task which involves extensive discussion as part of the activity. Expressing one's opinion on a given issue is built into the actual task. In this case, the therapist may be more involved during the activity to make sure all of the members participate and express their views and that their responses to one another are respectful and courteous.

Processing

This is often the most difficult step for students to learn. Inexperienced group leaders often skip this step entirely. Processing involves expressing how members feel about the experience, the leader and each other. Feelings guide our behavior more than we know, and they certainly influence patients' behavior in occupational therapy groups. If these emotions remain unexpressed, the outcome of the group can never be fully understood. Expressing feelings is not so difficult when the experience has been positive. But if there are negative feelings, people often wish to avoid expressing them, and this includes both the group members and the leader.

If done correctly, processing can reveal some important and relevant information. If members felt anxious, embarrassed or belittled while doing an activity, this will help to explain some of their responses when sharing and discussing it. Perhaps they felt intimidated by the leader, or angry with some of the other members. Feelings like this can override any possible benefit the activity may have, if they are not expressed before the group ends. When they are expressed, the therapist has the opportunity to incorporate them into the subsequent discussion and to help the patients understand the significance of the feelings related to the group experience.

Processing also includes a discussion of the non-verbal aspects of group. Underlying issues, such as struggles for power and control, subgrouping, scapegoating, conflict, attraction and avoidance, are dynamics that may never be verbalized, but will have a powerful influence on the group. These issues are highly complex for the beginning student; however, they should be well understood by the beginning therapist. Underlying dynamics such as those mentioned can and do occur naturally in all groups. They will strongly influence the outcome of our occupational therapy groups, both positively and negatively, and must be handled openly and skillfully. More will be discussed about the underlying process of groups in a later chapter.

Generalizing

This step addresses the cognitive learning aspects of the group. Here the therapist mentally reviews the group's responses to the activity, and tries to sum them up with a few general principles. If the activity has gone as expected, some of the general principles derived from the group should closely resemble the original goals. However, few groups go exactly as planned. The general principles discussed in the group should not be preplanned, but should come directly from the response of the members.

For example, an occupational therapist did an activity called "Incomplete Sentences" with a group of emotionally disturbed adolescents. The goal of the group was to clarify their values, and in fact, the group did accomplish this. However, some additional principles were brought up during the processing phase, which are important to note.

Principles of the "Incomplete Sentences" group:
1) The members generally value making decisions independent of their parents.
2) The most valued activities were those the members chose to do themselves, such as sleeping late on Saturdays or buying their own clothes.
3) Although wishing to be independent, members generally needed and wanted to be accepted by their parents as autonomous adults.

The third principle is the one not planned. During the processing phase, a member pointed out how good it was to be able to ask the leader to complete the sentences too. The group felt positive toward this leader, who, unlike their parents, seemed to accept them as equals. The comment brought forth many spontaneous stories of parental non-acceptance and it was evident that this was the important issue for the group.

General principles may be arrived at in several ways. The leader can look at the patterns of response among members. What opinions do they have in common? What were the common elements of their drawings or stories? For example, a group of alcoholics may see their drinking as the obstacle to reaching their vocational ambitions; bottles or glasses may appear in their drawings, or they may talk about highly unrealistic vocational ambitions. These common elements are easily seen as general principles. Another way to distinguish general principles is to look at areas of disagreement. What are the conflicted areas in the group? Some members, for example, may see stress as a motivator to get moving, while others may find it overwhelming and the cause of their inaction.

A third important clue to the general principles is the group's energy. The therapist should follow up on issues that seem to energize the group and stimulate spontaneous conversation. An example is the third principle in the "Incomplete Sentences" activity mentioned earlier. This is one of those unpredictable aspects of groups that makes them continually exciting and interesting.

Application

The application phase closely follows the generalizing phase, but takes it one step further. The therapist helps the group to understand how the principles learned during the group can be applied to everyday life. The goal is for each member to understand how he will apply the results of this group experience to help make his own life more functional outside the group.

To begin this process, the therapist should attempt to verbalize the meaning or significance of the experience; i.e., "Now that we know how important it is to have our parents' respect and acceptance, each of us needs to find a way to communicate this need to our parents." Application answers the question, "Now that you know how things are, what are you going to do about it?"

The answer to this question will be different for each individual. Knowledge of the patient's background is helpful. The therapist discusses with each member how the principles learned in the group relate to problems or issues each has expressed earlier. For example, Sue will have a hard time explaining to her father, who thinks of her as a child, that she needs for him to trust her judgment about whom she dates and where she goes on Saturday nights. Laura, whose mother travels extensively on business, will have difficulty just getting her mom's attention long enough to talk about it. She sometimes wonders if her mother cares about her enough to take the time. Both girls will have difficulty in communicating with their parents, but in very different ways. Application may sometimes resemble a kind of group problem solving members help each other find ways to apply the newly learned information.

One way the therapist can help the group with application is through limited self-disclosure. The therapist can role model application by saying, "When I need to discuss something with my mother and there never seems to be a good time, sometimes I suggest we make a date to go out to dinner together. She has to eat anyway and so do I, so that plan works well for both of us. How do you see that?" The self-disclosure is not so personal as to be distracting, but offers a possible method of getting parents' attention for the group to consider. It gives the group a concrete example and opens the door for them to make their own suggestions.

Summary

The final phase of the seven step group is the summary. The purpose of the summary is to verbally emphasize the most important aspects of the group so that they will be understood correctly and remembered. Like generalizing, there is really no way to pre-plan a summary. The points to emphasize should come directly from the group's responses. A good summary may take four or five minutes. It reviews the goals, the content and the process of the group. Sometimes the therapist asks the group members to help summarize by remembering the activity and giving their ideas about what was learned. The general principles are almost always included in the summary. Having members explain their own views of the group and how it can be applied, often reinforces the learning that took place.

The emotional content of the group is also important to summarize. Especially when the group feels positive or the mood has changed for the better, verbal recognition of the good feelings by the therapist will help members remember the group as a positive experience.

One way for the therapist to acknowledge feelings is to thank the members for their participation in the group. While this is not a formula, addressing and thanking individuals for their openness, honesty and willingness to share or trust in the group is always welcomed.

A final responsibility of the therapist is to end the group on time. If the group is well planned and lead, this will mark the completion of all seven steps. If, for some reason, all the steps have not been completed by the end of the session, the missing parts and the reasons for this can also be dealt within the summary.

Before leaving the "how to" section, three additional factors of leadership need to be explored: group motivation, limit setting and leadership styles. All are the responsibility of the leader and should occur throughout the seven steps as they are needed.

Group Motivation

Ideally, the therapist will have a group that comes to meetings with enthusiasm and interest to participate. Such a group will be eager to listen to the therapist and take direction. A group that is motivated will interact freely with one another, will share with one another easily and will spontaneously seek to know the meaning of the group activity and how it can be applied. Such a group is probably too healthy to need therapy. Therefore, the leader needs to develop skills in how to motivate groups that may not be so eager.

An important factor in the group's motivation is its confidence in the leader. If the leader takes charge of the group with some authority and sounds like he or she knows what to do, the leader will inspire the group's confidence and trust. This confidence is further enhanced by the support and encouragement offered to the members. If patients feel that the therapist empathizes with them and understands their situation, they will tend to be more cooperative in accepting leadership. Trust is the important issue here. Patients need to feel that the leader is sensitive to them and that he or she can and will respond to their needs. They also need to know the leader is in control in order to feel safe.

A leader also motivates the group members by encouraging *their* enthusiasm. This can be done in a number of ways. First, the leader can show enthusiasm for the group both verbally and non-verbally. A leader who smiles and speaks in a lively tone, makes frequent eye contact and demonstrates energetic movements often passes on enthusiasm to the group. Talking to members individually and encouraging them to participate may be effective. The approach to patients has to be adapted to the cognitive level of the patients. An explanation of how the group will make a difference in their lives will work for higher level patients. A more immediate benefit may need to be offered to lower functioning patients, i.e., "Doing this activity will make you feel more relaxed." Activities such as games or creative efforts chosen for the group may stimulate enthusiasm. Some activities will have built-in rewards, i.e., cooking groups and craft groups.

A final motivating factor is encouraging group interaction. It has been said that people get as much out of a group activity as they put into it. When group members are interacting with one another, they are not only participating, but also taking over some of the responsibility for the group. Interaction should be encouraged, especially in the sharing, processing, generalizing and application phases of the group. A good leader allows the group members to share the leadership to the extent that they are capable. If they can support one another during sharing, express how they feel about one another during processing, notice similarities and differences during generalizing and offer ideas to each other about application, they will then learn a lot more than if the leader does all these things for them. The leader can get the group to interact by indirectly encouraging them, or by asking them to do so directly, i.e., the leader might ask, "Susan, what do you think of Peter's drawing?" or "Peter, what do you think the group had in common?" Often, the leader only needs to ask questions a few times in order for the group to understand what is expected.

A leader who does all the talking in this seven stage group is working too hard. It benefits both the leader and the group by getting the group to talk more. Members who interact, respond and ask questions are showing their enthusiasm and helping others to become enthusiastic also. With the leader's guidance, the group can help accomplish many of its goals through interaction.

Setting Limits

This has to do with how the leader exerts authority over the group. The goal is to achieve a balance between control and leniency. The leader should *assume appropriate authority*, guiding the group through all its stages, while giving members the freedom to express their thoughts, feelings and opinions. A good leader will guide the group assuredly, but will not dominate or intimidate its members. Neither does a good leader allow him or herself to be dominated by the group. If the group goes its own way unguided, the members will not learn and make therapeutic change, and the group may never reach its goals.

Another part of setting limits is allowing sufficient time for each member to contribute. There are always a few members of a group who seem to take up more time and attention than the others. It is up to the therapist to see that all the members have a chance to participate. The leader controls the pace of the group and lets members know when they are taking more than their share of the time available. In this way, the group can be guided through each stage and can end on time.

Limiting inappropriate behavior is perhaps the most difficult for students to learn. It generally requires that the leader interrupt the process going on in order to request that it be changed. If Joe has embarked on a lengthy discussion about a staff member who has treated him unfairly, but the issue has nothing to do with the goals of the group, it may be necessary for the leader to stop him and redirect the group back to the task at hand.

Limits are best set with respect, and without anger, so that the group members won't become defensive. The therapist should develop skill in empathizing with the offending patient. When the leader asks Joe to stop his tirade about the staff member, it is more likely to be heard if he or she first acknowledges his anger: "Joe, it sounds like you're very angry at _____, and I'd be happy to listen to you tell me about it after the group. But for now, I'd like to hear what all the members have to say about leisure planning." Other types of inappropriate behavior might be members showing disrespect for or disinterest in one another, or physical expressions of emotion.

One important principle to keep in mind is *always* put the good of the group first. When individuals behave in ways that distract the group from benefiting in an occupational therapy activity, the leader is obligated to intervene on behalf of the group. Techniques for dealing with specific patient behaviors that are difficult will be discussed in the next chapter.

Leadership Styles

The leadership style a therapist uses will profoundly effect the outcome of the group. Furthermore, different frames of reference require very different leadership approaches. Knowing the characteristics of several approaches and their likely effects on the group, allows us to be flexible and use our skills more effectively to achieve desired outcomes.

According to Lewin (1938, 1939), there are three fundamental leadership styles: autocratic, democratic and laissez-faire. Autocratic leadership implies complete control of the group with little or no input from the members. Democratic leadership allows members to make choices and to have a say in what the group does and becomes. Laissez-faire is a French expression meaning literally "to let do" or to let the people do as they choose. Laissez-faire leadership implies a minimum of control and a deliberate non-interference in the natural forces of a group or the freedom of individuals within it. Lewin studied the effects of these three styles of leadership at a boys summer camp. He found that autocratic leadership resulted in the greatest productivity, but created hostility and resentment, poor quality of work and dependency on the leader. Laissez-faire leadership produced independence in the members, but morale was not very high. It was democratic leadership that resulted in the highest morale and the most group cohesiveness. However, Lewin's study should be understood in the context of the boys' camp. The democratic style that worked best for campers, may not work for other populations of subjects, and other styles may be more appropriate.

Three types of occupational therapy group leaderships will be presented in this text: director, facilitator and advisor. All may be defined democratic in spirit, but with varying amounts of member input. Each is appropriate in different situations, and for different levels of patient functioning.

Directive Leadership

In politics, an autocratic leader rules a dictatorship; he fashions the nation according to his own vision, setting up the structures of government and making all the decisions. In therapy, it would not ethical or desirable to hold this much control over a group of patients. However, as a director, the occupational therapist defines a group, selects activities and structures the group in ways which he or she knows to be therapeutically appropriate for a specific group of patients. The director used authority sparingly, only as necessary to make the group therapeutic for its members. Used inappropriately, too much direction can cause members to feel infantilized, treated like children who cannot think for themselves; it can stunt the growth and development of a group by crushing attempts to question or challenge the leader.

However, directive leadership is absolutely necessary for the lower functioning patients who do not have the cognitive capabilities to make decisions or solve problems. These patients do not feel safe when the therapist is not in control. In a sense, the therapist is always in control, even in the more democratic approaches. The leader sets the goals, the level of structure, the media used and the extent to which leadership responsibilities are shared with the group. The therapist's decisions about how to lead are hopefully, based not only on his or her own preference or style, but on the therapist's expert assessment of the needs of the group. For example, Allen suggests that the therapist structure the environment and the task demand, but within that context, allow patients to do as much as they can for themselves (Allen 1985). If the therapist is knowledgeable about Allen's theory, he or she will be able to predict fairly accurately how much assistance the patients will need to accomplish a task, and will plan the structure of the group accordingly.

Facilitative Leadership

The next style of leadership on the control vs. freedom continuum is democratic. Just as the democratic leader is voted into power by the citizens, a facilitator gathers support from constituents. The leader must convince the members of the group that he or she is on their side and represents their best interests. The facilitator earns the support of the members by allowing them to make choices, and showing care and concern. Decisions are made by the group with the facilitator's guidance. The therapist is a resource person, providing the group with needed information, needed structure and needed equipment and supplies. The OT facilitator openly discusses the purpose and goals of the group. Just as a democratic government presumes and requires a certain level of education in its citizens in order to work effectively, democratic leadership in therapy requires that the members have a certain level of knowledge and skill. Without the required knowledge, members cannot make good decisions or share the leadership effectively. So the role of a facilitator is also that of an educator. The therapist explains the therapeutic aspects of activity so that the group can choose tasks that are likely to be of benefit to them.

Lewin said that democratic leadership is the most likely to lead to group cohesiveness. This is confirmed in reviewing the group developmental process. (further described in Chapter 2). As a group reaches the "control" phase, they must challenge the leadership, the structure and the group task. A facilitator can allow herself to be challenged, use reason and logic to explain the way things have been, and give the group choices about changing them in ways that are not destructive to the group's integrity.

Group facilitation also has it's limitations. It is not suitable for patients functioning at a low cognitive level. It presumes a certain level of self-awareness, intelligence and insight or self-understanding. It is most useful in frames of reference which make personal direction and choice a priority. The humanistic, psychoanalytic (ego functions) and model of human occupation approaches depend on a facilitative leadership style to facilitate a certain level of independent functioning and decision-making in patient group members. However, when the goals of treatment are to develop specific skills and abilities or to promote neurophysiological or cognitive development, a democratic approach may not be appropriate.

Facilitation is the most useful in motivating patients and getting them involved. It is a widely recognized phenomenon that people tend to be more committed to pursuing goals which they have a part in choosing. The more cognitively aware they are, the more they resent goals that are imposed on them. Therefore, discussions which precede a group may use a facilitative approach as a motivator, even when the group itself is more directive.

Group Leader as Advisor

The advisor is the most passive of leadership styles. Its use in therapy is limited to the most high functioning groups working on goals like problem solving or attitude change. An OT leader/advisor may be appropriate in prevention or health maintenance. Clients who seek assistance with specific problems may need an occupational therapist to advise them on issues such as coping with stress on the job, conserving energy in the home, or eliminating architectural and social barriers. The advisor offers expertise as needed or requested, but does not provide structure or goals. Motivation comes from the group itself, and change is produced intrinsically as a result of the internal processes of each member. Frames of reference for which advisor leadership is most appropriate are psychoanalytic, humanistic and the model of human occupation.

General Principles of Therapy Group Leadership

Leaders of therapy groups, whatever their particular style, have certain obligations to the group. Designing the group is the most obvious of these. This planning phase involves choosing the members, setting or acknowledging the goals, setting the time and place, organizing the environment and choosing the activity or media (sometimes with help from members). The group protocol described in Chapter 10 serves as a guide for how to design a therapy group. Decisions about the best leadership style to use within a given patient setting are often complex. Table 1-1 may be helpful in choosing the best leadership style for certain member and activity characteristics.

Table 1-1.
Leadership Style Guidelines

Member Characteristics	Directive Leadership	Facilitative Leadership	Advisory Leadership
cognitive level	low	medium-high	high
insight capacity	minimal	fair-good	very good
group maturity	immature	medium-high	mature
verbal skills	poor	average	high
motivation	low	medium	high
Activity Characteristics			
structure	therapist selects activity	therapist and members select activity	members select activity
goals	accomplish task	learn skills from experience	understand process
instruction	therapist demonstrates/ teaches	therapist and members teach process	members seek advice as needed
group maintenance roles	mostly done by therapist	members share in leadership	members lead themselves
feedback	given mostly by therapist	members encouraged to give each other	natural consequences from environment

The ongoing functions of the leader are to help the group achieve its goals (task function) and to maintain the group's integrity (maintenance function). The therapist may need to focus the group on the task to prevent it from getting side-tracked. She may have to adapt the activity or task along the way. Maintaining the group can involve the use of many leader skills. Setting group norms, like confidentiality and mutual respect can be important. Modeling behaviors to be learned or effective interaction skills can help the group communicate and resolve its conflicts. The counselling skills Egan (1986) writes about are all useful in leading a therapeutic group: accurate empathy, concreteness, genuineness, confrontation and self-disclosure are examples. These are elaborated in Chapter 3. Giving members feedback and helping members to give and receive feedback is an important function of the leader. Keeping the communication channels open is vital to the survival and growth of groups. These norms and roles are elaborated in Chapter 2.

A Leadership Experience for Students

To practice the seven step group leadership, students may be divided into groups of eight to ten members. Each student should plan and lead a group of his or her peers for 45 minutes, followed by a 15 minute feedback session from the instructor (and members). Students who are beginning their professional training should not attempt to play the roles of patients. There are plenty of goals students will find useful to work on in these groups.

To help the student plan a group, the Practice Group Plan on the following page is suggested. The student's leadership skills may be evaluated by using the Leadership Evaluation worksheet.

Practice Group Plan

1. Title of Group

2. Purpose of the group

3. Brief description of activity

4. Supplies & equipment needed

5. Goals of the group

6. Questions for discussion in

   a) Processing

   b) Generalizing

   c) Application

7. Points for Summary

Leadership Evaluation Worksheet

Student Name: _____   Group Title: _____
Date: _____   Time: _____

Written Group Plan (10 points)

Introduction (10 points)

    Explains purpose clearly

    Asks for feedback from the group

    Uses warm-up to relax/prepare group

    Communicates expectations

    Outlines time frame/structure of group

Activity (10 points)

    Adequately prepared

    Directions clearly given

    Timing appropriate

    Materials appropriate

    Environment appropriate

Sharing (10 points)

    Invites each member to share

    Uses appropriate verbal and non-verbal communication

    Empathizes and acknowledges feelings of members

Processing (10 Points)

    Elicits members feelings about the experience

    Elicits members feelings about each other

    Elicits members feelings about the leader (when appropriate)

    Helps group understand its own processes

Generalizing (10 Points)

Points out like or similar responses

Points out contrasts or differences

Develops one or two principles learned

Group Motivation (10 Points)

Inspires confidence of group

Encourages enthusiasm

Encourages group interaction

Limit Setting (10 Points)

Allows sufficient time to each member

Limits inappropriate behavior

Assumes appropriate authority (but not too controlling)

Application (10 Points)

Verbalizes meaning of this experience (significance)

Shows how this experience can relate to everyday life

Relates this experience issues/problems of members

Uses concrete examples and/or self-disclosure

Summary (10 Points)

Chooses most important points to emphasize

Verbally reinforces group learning

Acknowledges contributions of members

Ends group on time

Member Evaluation Summary

Total Leadership Score:

Summary of Strengths:

Summary of Weaknesses:

Total Evaluation Score _____

Member Evaluation of Leader

Directions: This form may be used to obtain reactions of student members prior to discussion of student leader's performance in practice groups. The forms are then collected by the instructor and are considered when rating the student leader. Member evaluations are anonymous.

Date and time: Title of Activity:

How satisfied were you with the way the group was planned and led?

1. _____	2. _____	3. _____	4. _____	5. _____
Not at all satisfied	Somewhat satisfied	Satisfied	Very satisfied	Extremely satisfied

Please comment on how you found this group experience.

What did you see as the leader's strengths?

What did you see as the leader's weaknesses?

Conclusion

Although the seven steps are described without reference to theory, it should be noted that no approach is entirely atheoretical. The theoretical basis for this approach has some elements of the humanistic as well as the cognitive behavioral frames of reference. It has a sequence of steps that may be seen as developmental in their hierarchical order. These frames of reference (humanistic, cognitive behavioral and developmental) and their application to occupational therapy groups will be discussed in later chapters. The seven step approach is *not* intended to meet all needs for all patients. It can be adapted in many ways to reflect differing patients, goals and frames of reference.

Section Two will review several frames of reference occupational therapists have used to guide them in planning and leading groups. However, students often understand theory best when it relates to their experience. Therefore, it is suggested that students learn to lead groups first. They can practice their skills by leading groups of their peers. To accomplish this, a seven step sequence in leading groups has been described. This approach assumes a fairly high level of function among members. Members must be able to communicate with each other, trust and relate to each other and think abstractly. A high degree of cooperation and motivation is assumed. The approach is well-suited to college students, as well as physically disabled patients, substance abuse patients, patients with eating disorders and many other groups who are operating at a fairly high cognitive level.

Bibliography

Allen C. *Occupational Therapy for Psychiatric Diseases: Measurement and Management of Cognitive Disabilities.* Boston: Little Brown, 1985.

Johnson D. & Johnson F. *Joining Together: Group Theory and Group Skills.* 3rd ed. Englewood Cliffs, NJ: Prentice-Hall, 1987.

Lewin and Lippitt. *An Experimental Approach to the Study of Autocracy and Democracy: a Preliminary Note. Sociometry,* 1938, I, 292-300.

Lewin, Lippitt and White. Patterns of aggressive behavior in experimentally created social climates. *J of Social Psychology,* 1939, 10, 271-299.

Mosey A. *Occupational Therapy: Configuration of a Profession.* New York: Raven Press, 1982

Pfeiffer J. and Jones J. *Reference Guide to Handbooks and Annuals.* 2nd ed. La Jolla, CA.: University Associates, 1977.

Posthuma B. *Small Groups in Therapy Settings: Process and Leadership.* Toronto: Little, Brown & Co., 1989.

Raths L, Harmin M and Simon S. *Values and Teaching.* 2nd ed. Columbus, OH: Merrill, 1978.

Rider B. and Gramblin J. *The Activity Card File.* 1987. (available from Barbara Rider, O.T. Dept, Western Michigan University, Kalamazoo, MI, 49004).

Simmons P. and Mullins L. *Acute Psychiatric Care,* Thorofare, NJ: SLACK Incorporated, 1981.

Simon S., Howe L. and Kirschenbaum H. *Values clarification.* NY: A&W Publishers, 1972..

Stevens J. *Awareness.* Moab, Utah: Real People Press, 1971.

Understanding Group Dynamics

The large body of knowledge regarding group dynamics developed by behavioral scientists over the last fifty years offers a great deal of help in our understanding of how groups work. This body of knowledge comes from a variety of theoretical bases, the most common are humanistic, behavioral and psychoanalytic. Because of the verbal nature of the groups being researched, some assumptions have been made about the populations upon which these theories are based. Although even the most dysfunctional groups achieve some level of social organization, members of a group who have verbal skills and are capable of interaction can more easily demonstrate the **dynamics** described. Another assumption is that when there is enough freedom within the group structure for members to initiate and make choices, the dynamics will be more obvious. A third assumption is that the members are intrinsically motivated to self-improve through self-understanding and by increasing their interaction skills. All of these assumptions are similar to those in the existential/humanistic frame of reference in Chapter 3.

In general, group dynamics are the forces which influence the interrelationships of members and ultimately effect group outcome. It is important for occupational therapists to understand these forces when planning and implementing treatment groups. Groups have predictable stages of development and will respond best to different activities at different stages. As leaders, our recognition of our group's stage of development should influence our selection of activities. How we design and lead groups also depends on our recognition and understanding of the various dynamics. Some of the "dynamics" that will be included in this chapter are: group process, group development, leadership styles, norms and roles, special problems and termination.

Group membership experiences are emphasized in this chapter so that students can gain an appreciation for what patients might be experiencing under different group conditions. It is hoped that membership experiences will help occupational therapy students to be more observant and empathetic group leaders.

Group Process

We have already discussed processing as one step in group leadership. An awareness of the underlying process of groups is essential to our approach as therapists. It gives us many clues as to the feelings and motives of members and helps the therapist to make patients aware of these and their impact on wellness and on group function. Irvin Yalom has written a great deal about the process of psychotherapy groups.

Process is often first understood by what it is not. It is not content. The content of a group is what is done and what is said. For example, the group did pencil drawings and topics discussed were the jobs members had and how they liked them. Bob said he likes being a carpenter, but Sarah hates being a teacher. Process does not include past history or even recent history of the members. Its thrust is what is happening in the group, between and among members, right now. Process concerns the interpersonal relationship of the participants.

There are two parts to process in groups, according to Yalom: "If the powerful therapeutic factor of interpersonal learning is to be set into motion, the group must recognize, examine and understand process. It must study itself; it must study its own transactions; it must transcend pure experience and apply itself to the integration of that experience" (Yalom 1985, 136). So the process is experienced first, and then it "performs a self-reflective loop," examining what just occurred. The "processing" step in the preceding chapter, represents a simplified self-reflective loop (Figure 2-1). Members are asked to reveal how they felt about the activity they just experienced, as well as how they felt about the leader and each other. So the process commentary begins. Its emphasis is often on emotion and its purpose is to establish a cognitive framework that permits members to retain the group experience so that it can be generalized and applied.

The process comments are largely the responsibility of the therapist. He/she can and should request member participation, but he or she chooses the direction of intervention according to the needs of the group.

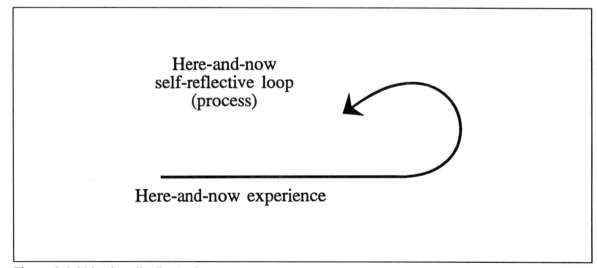

Figure 2-1. Yalom's self reflective loop.

Example

In a task group, the occupational therapist had taken considerable time in helping the group plan their next activity. They were going to construct kites. The plan for Monday was to walk to a craft store (about four blocks from the hospital) to buy paper, string, sticks and paint. The kites would be constructed during the next two sessions. The seven members of the group assembled with jackets, sneakers, etc. ready for the walk. Hannah, age 63, the eldest member of the group, was not feeling well, and refused to go. Dave, a 23-year-old member, bluntly asked the therapist if Hannah was too sick to walk. The reply was that she was fine medically. So Dave proceeded to call Hannah a "lazy do-nothing complainer." The other members verbally attacked Dave for his rudeness and insensitivity to the elder member, and a heated argument ensued until it was too late to carry out the plan.

Content

As an occupational therapy leader, how would you process this group? First, it is helpful to identify content. What was the overt experience? The group came prepared to walk to the craft store as planned. The plan was not carried out because Hannah refused to go. What was verbalized? Dave was verbally abusive to Hannah. The other members verbally attacked Dave for being abusive, and he defended himself with counter attacks, shouting loudly at the group. The virtues of courtesy to one's elders was discussed.

Process

The process involves what is implied by the content. The therapist might consider the following possibilities.

1) Hannah wanted some attention and chose to pursue it by her passivity. Perhaps her refusal was her way of exerting control over the group, or perhaps illness is her usual way of getting attention.
2) The other group members were frustrated at not being able to carry out their plan, and were looking for someone to blame.
3) Hannah was to blame, but she seemed too frail and vulnerable to be verbally accused.
4) Dave was impatient and expressed his frustration aggressively. Perhaps aggressive-ness is his usual way of coping with frustration, a habit that often gets him in trouble; or perhaps he feels guilt and is looking for a way to be punished.
5) The group's frustration, diverted from Hannah by her vulnerability, was vented on Dave instead. Dave was made the scapegoat of the group. A **scapegoat** is something which symbolizes all the badness of the group or someone who is blamed for its problems. The scapegoat generally serves the purpose of allowing the group to avoid its own responsibility for what has occurred.
6) Perhaps the group wanted to avoid either the walk or the activity. Dave and Hannah gave them an excuse to avoid doing any task-oriented problem solving.

Needs to be Addressed

Which hypothesis is correct? Any or all of them are. How, then, should the therapist intervene to help the group understand its process? The first thing a leader should ask herself is "what does this group really need?" Here are some possible needs to be addressed:

1) The foremost need is to get Dave off the "hot seat." He may have been rude and aggressive, making him an easy target for the group, but he is certainly not the direct cause of their frustration. If Dave is not rescued, he will probably be forced

out of the group, and will be left feeling angry and hurt. Being scapegoated is not a therapeutic experience.

For Dave, the therapist might point out how his behavior tends to elicit this kind of response from others, and how he set himself up to be the scapegoat. For the members of the group, the therapist might discuss their feelings about Hannah. They need to understand why they avoided blaming her, how they ended up in a struggle with Dave and what they themselves were avoiding by pursuing the argument.

2) The therapist might then want to examine the issue of Hannah's control. What are her real needs (attention, respect) and how might they be pursued more appropriately? An awareness of her pattern of controlling others with her illness, real or otherwise, might be very helpful as a beginning step toward therapeutic change. The group's collusion with her in achieving her goal to keep the group from acting is another important issue. Why did they allow her to exert such control? What purpose did it serve for them? Why did they not exclude her instead of Dave?

3) The final issue of importance is the group's relationship to the task. How did they feel about the activity they chose? Were they really that invested? Or were they looking for an excuse not to pursue it? What were the group's choices? Could they have found an alternative way to get their supplies? Could they have reorganized their roles so that Hannah would not have to go on the walk, without excluding her from the group as a whole? If walking is important to them in getting out of the hospital to enjoy the spring weather, perhaps Hannah could have been wheeled in a wheelchair, or she could have walked part of the way and then waited with another member.

If the group is to learn from this rather frustrating and upsetting experience, it is evident that they need the occupational therapist's guidance in problem-solving. Finding alternative solutions and compromising are essential if the group is to accomplish its task. Steps should be taken before the end of this group to avoid a reoccurrence of frustration in the next session.

Discovering the Process of Groups

The best way for students to learn about group process is to experience it. Therefore, a real example taken from a student group experience is best used for this exercise. However, if that is not available, the student may use the following example. Use the Content-Process Reaction Worksheet to evaluate the experience.

The group was engaged in doing an assertiveness exercise. All the members had anonymously written down situations on a card, and put them in a basket in the center of the table. Members had to draw a card, read it and tell what they would do to assertively handle the situation described on the card. Mary drew a card and read it to the group. It said "On my fieldwork experience, I was working with two patients and one of them started to cry. I didn't know why she was crying so I ran down the hall to find a nurse, leaving the two patients alone in the clinic. I couldn't believe that my supervisor, Miss Hunt, failed me for leaving the patients alone." Mary looked bewildered. "How could the supervisor expect you to know what to do? You're just a student." Maureen, another member said, "How could the student be so stupid? If she doesn't know what to do, she shouldn't be in occupational therapy." Susan added, "But I had Miss Hunt too. She's really a hard nose." Several others commented on Miss Hunt's inadequacy as a supervisor. Laurie agreed with Maureen, "Yes, but the student should have known better." Roberta listened silently to this debate, looking more and more distressed as the end of the session approached.

Content-Process Reaction Worksheet

Directions: Write the answers to these questions after you have participated in the group session.

 I. Content
   A. Give a brief description of the activity.

   B. Identify three major participants and what topics they discussed. If there were more than three, choose the three you think were most important.
     1) Person:
        Topic:
        Others Offering Feedback:
        Approximate Length of Time:
     2) Person:
        Topic:
        Others Offering Feedback:
        Approximate Length of Time:
     3) Person:
        Topic:
        Others Offering Feedback:
        Approximate Length of Time:

II. Process
   A. Name three feelings you personally experienced during the group. To whom/ what were the feelings directed?
     1)
     2)
     3)

   B. Based on your observations of verbal and non-verbal behavior, what are some hypotheses (possible explanations or interpretations) about the process of the group?
     1)
     2)
     3)
     4)
     5)

   C. Based on the above hypotheses, what therapeutic intervention(s) would you make as a leader and why?

Group Development

Group development refers to the stages groups go through as they progress from initiation to termination. Several theorists have contributed to this aspect of groups, including Schutz, Bion, Tuckman and Yalom (Table 2-1). Knowing the characteristics of each stage helps the therapist know what to expect. It helps him/her predict how the group will respond to certain activities, and therefore plan appropriately.

Research shows that all groups progress through a series of predictable stages. Many theories have been suggested as to what these stages are, and in fact, all seem to have similar characteristics. There is an initial stage of orientation, with its search for structure, goals and dependency on the leader. Next, there is a stage of conflict with its struggle for dominance and rebellion against the leader. Then there is a growth of interpersonal harmony and intimacy, sometimes called cohesiveness. The final outcome is a mature working group characterized by high cohesiveness and commitment to the goals of the group-therapeutic learning.

Our knowledge of group development comes from a collection of studies including observations of therapy groups, training groups (educational), natural groups and laboratory groups.

Table 2-1.
Summary of Group Development Theories

	Stage 1	Stage 2	Stage 3	Stage 4
Tuckman (1965)	Forming	Storming	Norming	Performing
Bion (1961)	Flight	Fight	Unite	
Schutz (1958)	Inclusion	Control	Affection	
Yalom (1985)	Orientation	Conflict	Harmony	Maturity

Tuckman

Tuckman (1965) published the first major review of these studies from which he abstracted a theory of four stages of group development: 1) forming, 2) storming, 3) norming and 4) performing. Tuckman believed that all the stages occur in some way regardless of the duration of the group, i.e., shorter length groups impose the requirement of the problem-solving stages to be reached quickly; therefore, the rate of development tends to adjust to the time available.

Tuckman's initial stage, **forming**, involves orientation and testing regarding the group task and a dependence on the leader for guidance. **Storming** involves conflict among group members as they challenge the task, the rules and the leader. In the **norming** stage harmony prevails and members accept and trust one another while conflicts are avoided. The last stage, **performing** goes beyond cohesiveness to a point where conflict can be openly discussed and resolved. A performing group can effectively work together in a supportive emotional environment that encourages growth and therapeutic change.

Bion

Bion's work is also frequently quoted, especially with the easy-to-remember titles of the stages: 1) flight, 2) fight and 3) unite. Bion (1961) looked at the behavior of groups at conferences, having a task rather than a therapeutic focus. **Flight** represents an avoidance of some problem or threat. Members tend to turn to each other in pairs for more intimate emotional response in this stage. The **fight** stage represents the challenge of the leader (and possibly scapegoating a rival member-leader). **Uniting** follows these two emotional states; it settles down the members to a stable working group with relatively little emotionality. Bion's work, although emerging from the corporate and industrial arena has many parallels in the therapeutic group. This may be especially applicable to the occupational therapy group which, although therapeutic in its goal, tends to be more task focused.

Schutz

Schutz's (1958) theory, while similar to those previously described, tends to have the clearest interpersonal focus. He says that every individual has three interpersonal needs: inclusion, control and affection. These needs parallel those of a child in the family, and are generalized to any interpersonal relationship among two or more individuals. In other words, groups follow the same sequence of interpersonal concerns as individuals do. Schutz's stages are shown to have both individual and group characteristics.

Inclusion Stage

In the inclusion stage, the individual is concerned with being accepted: "where do I fit in? Will I be important? respected? Can I be myself? How will the leader respond to me?" The group behaviors observed are: overtalking, attention seeking, territoriality and individual self-centeredness. Members listen but don't really hear what others say. They tend to look to the leader when they speak rather than each other. In this initial phase the rational approach is dominant; emotions do not flow freely. The group explores the goals, rationale and structure. The leader is looked to for the answers. There are multiple attempts at sizing each other up. Members look for similarities and tend to downplay differences. There is concern over those who haven't made a contribution, and rightly so. For if members are continually passive, they can become blockers to the progress of the group as a whole.

Control Stage

Schutz's control stage also has individual and group concerns. The individual now questions "Where do I stand in relation to power and authority? How much influence do I have? Will I have too much responsibility?" The group is generally at some point, engaged in a leadership struggle. The once "all powerful and all knowing leader" (therapist) is now viewed with skepticism and mistrust.

If the leader abdicates, that is, gives up the leadership, a struggle among members ensues to fill the void. Scapegoating of a would-be leader is common, and attempts to lead are often met with severe criticism, or are ignored. Members often disagree about how much structure is needed, or how the group should be led, and sub-groups may arise. There is ambivalence about the leader, like a two-year-old child, the group at once wants to be autonomous but needs the leader's support and protection.

The importance of all this for occupational therapists is in knowing that rebellion and challenge among group members is *normal* and *necessary* to the healthy development of the group. Be prepared to be challenged, and don't take it as a personal affront. How then, should we as occupational therapists handle the challenge? There are three choices. 1) An advisor as leader would tend to back down, to abdicate leadership. To do so invites intragroup conflict which could be more stressful than patients can handle. 2) A director would subdue the rebellion. In this case the therapist remains the leader and encourages further dependency of the group. Such an approach has been known to stifle group development. 3) The democratic leader would not abdicate all the control, but would encourage the group to share the leadership. This is Yalom's approach. He states that the group needs to experience the freedom and the responsibility for the group outcome. He suggests the leader not abdicate, but allow expression of dissension and acknowledge it. The therapist should "take the blows" and not allow any group members to become a scapegoat. Ideally, the therapist will make some changes in response to the group to allow the conflict to resolve while preserving the integrity of the group.

Affection Stage

If the conflict in leadership is resolved successfully, the group progresses to the affection stage. This is the stage of group cohesiveness, when attention focuses on "How do others feel about me?" and then "How do we feel about each other?" The group is characterized by expression of positive feeling and emotional investment in the group. Members are able to really listen to each other and even direct hostility may be expressed without devastating consequences.

The affection stage is the goal for any therapy group. Here is where members feel safe, cherished and trusting in one another. This allows members to explore new behaviors and to grow. They value one another, and therefore, they value themselves. There is real altruism and real consensual validation; members want to help each other and accept feedback from each other to validate their own self-perceptions. It is part of our role, as occupational therapists, to help our groups to reach this stage.

Nevertheless, there are some real barriers to achieving the affection stage. Schutz tells us that groups tend to regress easily, even after they have reached this stage. Events such as the arrival of a new member, leaving of an old member, leadership changes and long holidays will all cause a group to regress. Furthermore, patients who are lacking in social and interpersonal skills and/or who are unable to trust others, may be incapable of reaching the affection stage. Anticipation of termination of the group inevitably causes the development to reverse. A cohesive group may sink, once again, into conflict in preparation for breaking the ties and moving on.

How Groups Reach Maturity

Why should OT's study group development? There are several reasons. First, understanding the progression to maturity in groups gives us something to strive for; it shows us what is the true capacity of a mature, cohesive group. As therapists we should do whatever we can to help the group reach a mature, working stage. Corey (1988) suggests one way to speed up the process is to prepare members to get the most from a group. Corey's guidelines are helpful to students participating in a group lab and may be kept in mind as suggestions for our higher functioning patients. Some of the suggestions are summarized as follows:

Have a Focus

Think about what you'd like to get from the group, what issues you'd like to explore and changes you'd like to make. Writing down your goals prior to each group is often helpful.

Pay Attention to Feelings

Groups are an opportunity to explore personal issues that are often heavily laden with emotion. It is often the emotions that emerge that offer important insights and an opportunity for personal growth. The group is not a place to censor expression of emotions, but rather to let them flow. Feelings that are bottled up session after session, will eventually "dam up the flow of the group" (Corey 1988, 48).

Be an Active Participant

"You will help yourself most if you take an active role in the group. Silent observers are not as likely to get as much from their participation in the group, and others may believe their silence means they are being judgmental" (Corey 1988, 48).

Give Feedback

Whether positive or negative, your honest and direct response to others will move the group toward a deeper level of trust. Occupational therapists look forward to a long career of giving constructive feedback to patients. It is essential for occupational therapy students to develop the skill of giving honest feedback in ways that are empathetic and respectful of the other member.

Be Open to Feedback

Others in the group may not have perfected the art of giving constructive feedback. When someone responds honestly but bluntly, it is natural to get defensive in justifying your own standard and therefore to reject their feedback. Instead of letting defenses sabotage your work in the group, use the group as an opportunity to discover your defenses, which might include "rationalizing, withdrawing, denying, or turning a specific criticism into a global 'I'm no good'"(Corey 1988, 51). Try to get beyond your defenses and learn to use feedback constructively.

Take Responsibility for What You Accomplish

It is easy to blame others when you're bored, annoyed or unable to self-disclose in the group. Take a look at your own contribution to this state of affairs and instead of blaming the group, think about what you could do to make things better. You have a great deal of control and choice about how you interact with others in the group, and in the final analysis, what you accomplish is up to you. Corey's suggestions are some individual behaviors and beliefs that can help groups move toward cohesiveness. We as occupational therapists, have many activities at our disposal that encourage the group to move in the direction of cohesiveness. An example is the structured group activity called *Giving and Receiving Feedback* (Session 3 in Chapter 11).

Secondly, because the stages are predictable, knowledge of group development prepares us for what is coming next. It makes us better able to plan occupational therapy activities that are appropriate at each stage of development. For example, a "trust circle"exercise, requiring members to intentionally fall into the arms of other group members, and trust that they will be protected, may not be a good activity to introduce in the control stage of a group. Even the best laid plans might have to be changed because of changes in the stage of the group's development. For example, in a student training group, I had planned a structured exercise in setting priorities for the sixth session of the group. The group had developed beyond the control stage to a level of intimacy that made them almost cohesive. Sharing their priorities seemed too superficial so they rejected it and modified the activity to a discussion of how to rescue their troubled relationships. The group let me know very quickly that they needed to deal with something on a deeper level.

Another reason for studying group development is that the role of the leader changes with each stage. As occupational therapy leaders, we need to know what to expect. Imagine if you were a student leading a group and one week the patients all decided to rebel against you. Suppose you didn't know that this is a normal process for groups? How would you feel? One student leading time management group for substance abusers, was faced with a patient uprising. Quite unexpectedly, several members of the group refused to do the prescribed activity. Rather than forcing them to do it, she changed the agenda to a discussion of what they did and didn't like about the group. This student did not get defensive (fortunately) but listened intently to the patients' complaints and wrote down their suggestions. Group development theory had given this student some guidelines about how to handle the conflict. She knew she could not give up her leadership role, but neither was there any way she was going to force six grown men to do an activity they didn't want to do. By listening to them and taking them seriously, she allowed them to challenge her in a way that didn't threaten her and didn't threaten the integrity of the group either. The following week they were able to approach the activity (one they themselves had suggested) with renewed interest and enthusiasm.

Identifying Group Stages

A good way to learn about the stages of group development is to reflect on a group one has participated in for several sessions. If the group meets for ten weeks, the self-reflection about the stage of development should not start until at least the fifth session. If the stages are discussed too soon, before the conflicts begin, the discussion will not be meaningful.

Furthermore, too close a scrutiny will make the group self-conscious and therefore, inhibit its flow. The leader takes her cue from the group itself in the timing of a discussion of developmental stages.

As a self-learning tool, the student group member might look at the characteristics of each stage and see if these behaviors can be found in her group. Table 2-2 may be useful in assisting with this process. As behaviors are recognized, examples of these in one's own group may be cited. Generally, if three or four of the behaviors are present for a given stage, that one is likely to be correct. As an example, my student group lab was scheduled to do the *Giving and Receiving Feedback* exercise. Some of them questioned if they were ready for it. They claimed they didn't know each other well enough to say anything critical. They asked me to allow them to modify the activity so they wouldn't have to say anything negative. A few said, with hostility, they would just have to "make something up." A few others counter-attacked with the rationale that they would soon have to give constructive feedback to patients and this would give them some practice. I did not allow them to modify the activity but did allow them to vent their frustrations and fears and make their suggestions. Clarification and examples were given on how to give constructive feedback. The activity was carried out with a great deal of anxiety, but ending in relief when it was "not as hard as we thought."

Considering the above example, try the Group Development Evaluation.

Table 2-2.
Schutz's Stages of Development of Groups

I. Inclusion - behaviors
   1) Depend on leader to structure
   2) Look to leader for answers
   3) Rational approach dominates
      discuss topics/opinions/thoughts
      avoid feelings
      look for purpose/goals for group
   4) Individual behaviors predominate
      attention-getting or withdrawal
      humor/laughter
      territoriality/pairing
      talking but not listening
      referring back to prior experiences
   5) Search for similiarities
      energy is in keeping harmony
      find "what we agree on"
      avoid conflicts
   6) Concern over belonging/approval
      only say what will be accepted
      eye contact, verbalize mostly with leader
      seating changes frequently

II. Control - behaviors
   1) Ambivalence toward leader
      challenge structure/purpose
      challenge leader style
      challenge authority of leader
      test limits/rules
      need for leader protection/approval
   2) Disenchantment with group
      subgroups struggle among selves
      leader viewed with distrust
      members critical and discounting of group
   3) Sharing group responsibility
      dependence-independence struggle
      members share leadership functions
      suggestions for change in structure and task emerge
      member-leaders emerge
      competition, not cooperation, predominates
      leader bends will of group

III. Affection - behaviors
   1) Focus on feeling
      express feelings about each other
      express feelings about the leader
      consensual validation occurs
      direct hostility expressed constructively
   2) Delight in company of others
      identity with group
      feel one is lovable and loved
      concern that one is not lovable and not loved
      altruistic desire to help others
      separation anxiety
      new behaviors are explored

Group Development Evaluation

Directions: List six different behaviors or events in the group in the first column. Then in the second column, identify the stage of development in which this behavior would best be categorized.

Group Behaviors	Stage I, II or III
1.	
2.	
3.	
4.	
5.	
6.	

Stage of Development for this group is _____.

Group Norms and Roles

Norms

Norms are present in every group; they incorporate certain attitudes and standards of behavior that are acceptable to the group. Norms may be specified and verbalized by the leader, or they may not be verbalized but only implied by the behavior and interactions of members. The norms of a group may change as it develops or as members come and go. The therapist's awareness of the norms and their acceptance by the group helps him or her understand better the behaviors observed in the members.

The leader is responsible for establishing explicit ground rules for the group, like being on time and respecting the opinions of others. These are expectations the leader will announce at the outset and enforce as the group continues. Confidentiality has been mentioned earlier as a common explicit norm of groups. This means that what members say and do during group sessions should not be revealed or discussed with non-members. The agreement to keep group work confidential is an extension of the patient-therapist relationship: what patients say and do is considered privileged information. Knowing this, the patients can trust one another and are more likely to open up to the group.

Non-explicit norms are more elusive, because they are seldom verbalized. These may even be beyond the group's awareness. They may be understood in terms of behaviors that are acceptable or non-acceptable in the group. For example, the avoidance of conflict may be a norm in the beginning stages of groups. Certain topics may be considered taboo, to be discouraged or avoided. Norms develop in all groups, therapeutic or otherwise. Yalom points out that the norms of a therapy group are radically different from the rules of etiquette in social groups. In therapy, not only must members interact freely, they must also feel free to comment spontaneously on their immediate feelings about each other and the leader. Yalom describes the desirable norms of a therapy group as "active involvement in the group, non-judgmental acceptance of others, extensive self-disclosure, desire for self-understanding, dissatisfaction with present modes of behavior and eagerness for change (Yalom 1985, 117). These norms do not develop automatically. The leader uses considerable influence to shape the norms of a therapy group, with necessary help from its members.

Furthermore, the leader should closely monitor the non-explicit norms of the group. The adoption of non-therapeutic norms must be avoided at all costs, because once norms are established, they are very difficult to change. The therapist is the key influence in shaping norms. Yalom suggests that therapists do this in two ways: as a technical expert and as the model-setting participant.

As technical expert, the therapist relies on his/her experience and knowledge to introduce therapeutic norms and the reasons for them. Then, as the group goes on, the therapist may use social reinforcers to encourage the enactment of therapeutic norms, while discouraging anti-therapeutic norms. For example, one pattern that should be discouraged is the group members speaking only to the leader. We have already learned that dependence on the leader is a characteristic of the early stages of groups. A typical picture of this interaction is shown in Figure 2-2.

In the earliest stages, the leader establishes a norm of group interaction in several ways. He or she can refuse to answer the questions of members and reflect these to other members. For example, Mary asks the leader, "What are we supposed to talk about?" The leader does not answer, but responds with a question, "What might be some meaningful issues to talk about today?" As members begin to give their ideas, the therapist might ask,

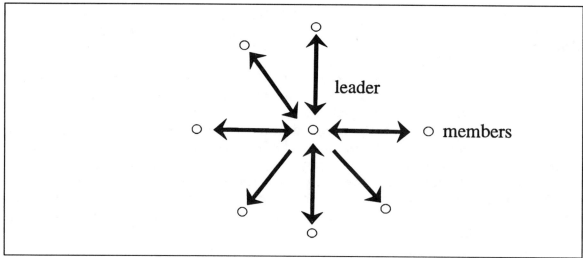

Figure 2-2. Leader-centered Interaction.

"Mary, what do you think about Sally's idea?" or "Sally, why don't you give Bill some feedback about his suggestion?" In this way, the leader tactfully establishes a communication pattern that looks more like Figure 2-3.

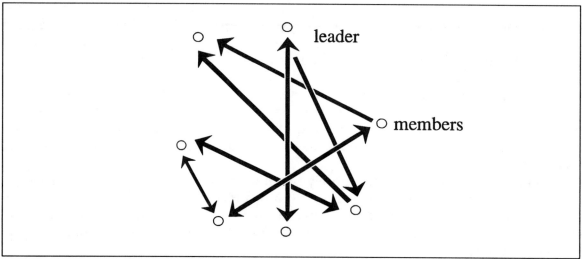

Figure 2-3. Group-centered Interaction.

Members are speaking not only to the leader, but addressing each other as well. This is an important norm to set in an interactive occupational therapy group, where members are expected to give each other feedback and learn from each other. This norm also helps the group to progress beyond the initial stage of development.

In this example, the therapist has used his or her role as both technical expert and model setting participant. The therapist has guided the group by telling them that they should interact with one another, and demonstrated the behaviors by asking specific group members to respond to one another.

Self-disclosure might be another way to model expected behaviors. When asking members to share their feelings, the leader may begin by sharing his or her own. Referring to the situation described earlier, the therapist might say: "When Maureen criticized the student for not knowing what to do with a patient who cried, I felt very concerned about how that student was feeling. Yet I was frustrated, because the situation was presented anonymously and I didn't know who wrote it. I didn't want to force this student to reveal herself, but I was afraid she would really be hurt and I wanted to protect her from the attack. I wonder if other members had some of these feelings also." This example demonstrates several expectations. The norm of free expression of emotion in the group is demonstrated by the leader's expression of both concern (fear) and frustration. The focus on "here and now" is demonstrated in the leader's encouragement of responses to one another within the group about what just occurred. The therapist's encouragement of concern for one another and not allowing members to criticize on another in a hurtful way, helps establish a norm of safety and trust. Finally, this self-disclosing comment invites the group to reflect on its own process, encouraging a norm of self-reflection in the group.

The norms in this example are some of what Yalom considers to be therapeutic norms. Some therapeutic norms Yalom refers to are: self-reflection of the group, encouraging self-disclosure, encouraging free interaction among members, reinforcing the importance of the group, regarding members as agents of change and setting an atmosphere of safety and support.

Norms will necessarily change in different groups. In occupational therapy groups, norms will vary with the patient populations we deal with and our frame of reference. Norms also change as the group moves through the stages of development. A comment which is unacceptable in stage one may be right on target in stage two or three. For example, the avoidance of conflict may be normal in stage one, but gives way to open criticism of the leader and the group structure in stage two. The norm of open conflict in turn gives way to a norm of acceptance of constructive feedback in stage three.

If a group is to progress in its development, norms must, from time to time, be challenged. Members who do so are considered to be taking a **risk**. Risks involve revealing yourself to the group in a way that makes you vulnerable, and taking the chance that you will be accepted and supported. In risks, there is always the chance that you may not get the response you're looking for. For example, after a very tense session in *Giving and Receiving Feedback*, Roberta shared with the group that she was rather hurt that someone in the group considered her to be aggressive and intimidating. Another member, Jennifer, took Roberta's cue and shared that she was confused by someone's comment that she was a snob, and "looked down her nose" at peers who weren't as smart as she was. The comments of Roberta and Jennifer were met with silence. Shortly afterward, the group ended.

What risks did Jennifer and Roberta take? How did the group respond? How do you think the group changed (or should change) as a result of their risk-taking behaviors? What norms did these two students challenge? Use the following worksheet to evaluate a group experience.

Monitoring Norms

As a learning exercise, write down the following after each group experience. Your comments can address many individual and group behaviors, but here are some suggestions: seating pattern, structure and format of the group, timing, silence, topics discussed, communication pattern, expression of emotion, discussion of process and leader intervention.

A. List three behaviors which were accepted by the group.

    1.

    2.

    3.

B. List three behaviors which were not (or would not be) accepted in this group.

    1.

    2.

    3.

C. List three expectations established by the leader.

    1.

    2.

    3.

D. List three of your own expectations for this group.

    1.

    2.

    3.

E. What norms have changed from the last group? Which norms would you like to see changed?

    1.

    2.

    3.

In considering the example of Roberta and Jennifer, it is clear that neither left the group happy. They were both angry and silent during the next group session. The group, left on its own, perhaps would have continued to ignore the behavior, which in some way threatened the group's status quo. In this case, the therapist has to make some judgment calls. Are Jennifer and Roberta mature and stable enough to handle the group's response or do they need support in continuing to take risks? Is the group ready to change its norms and open up to challenge and conflict? In the group exercise *Giving and Receiving Feedback* (Chapter 10, Session 3), the members' feedback to one another is anonymous. At what point are members ready to accept responsibility for their comments and give up the safety of anonymity? The leader's intervention should be protective of Roberta and Jennifer and supportive of their vulnerability, while being sensitive to the level of trust within the group. The best intervention, considering these factors, would be to use these members' risk-taking behaviors as a way of encouraging the silent members to take risks also. Only when the writers of the seemingly hurtful comments take the risk of revealing themselves, can the issues be discussed and resolved. Members can learn a great deal from this process, not the least of which is learning to give critical feedback in a caring and helpful way, and learning to accept critical feedback as an opportunity to grow and make therapeutic change.

Roles

Roles are the result of the members dividing the work of the group among themselves. Members play roles such as follower, initiator, energizer and blocker, spontaneously as the group progresses, or roles may be assigned by the leader. Researchers have identified the more frequent roles played in groups, and have organized these according to their functions. Some roles tend to help the group accomplish a task, while others help maintain the group's lines of communication. Still other roles tend to interfere with group function, such as an attention seeker or a monopolist. The therapist not only needs to recognize these roles, she should help members take on a variety of roles, and to change those roles which are detrimental to the group. It is often through taking on different roles that much of the therapeutic learning takes place in the group setting.

The concept of group roles was introduced in 1948 by two researchers, Kenneth Benne and Paul Sheats. Their idea was to look at leadership of the group not as solely present in the identified leader or therapist, but as a shared responsibility of all the members. These writers suggest that "the quality and amount of group production is the 'responsibility' of the group ...(and) the setting of goals and the marshalling of resources to move toward these goals is a group responsibility in which all members of a mature group come variously to share" (Cathcart and Samovar 1974, 180). Benne and Sheats developed from their research at the National Training Lab in Group Development in 1947, their now classic breakdown of member roles into 1) group task roles, 2) group building and maintenance roles and 3) individual roles.

A group role is a behavior pattern or structured way of behaving within the group. Group roles tend to remain stable regardless of who is in them. Thus, a single group member can take on a variety of roles within the group, and members can change their roles as often as they wish. Since there is a relationship between personality and the roles one typically plays with others, the roles members find themselves taking on can, in itself, be revealing. However, the roles themselves are interchangeable. Maturity has been measured by the ability to take on a variety of group roles.

Task Roles

These are the roles which help the group to get its work done. There are twelve:

1. Initiator-contributor - suggests new ideas, innovative solutions to problems, unique procedures and new ways to organize
2. Information seeker - asks for clarification of suggestions, focusing on facts
3. Opinion seeker - seeks clarification of values and attitudes presented
4. information giver - offers facts or generalizations "automatically"
5. Opinion giver - states beliefs or opinions
6. Elaborator - spells out suggestions and gives examples
7. Coordinator - clarifies relationships among various ideas
8. Orienter - defines position of group with respect to its goals
9. Evaluator-critic - subjects accomplishments of group to some standard of group functioning
10. Energizer - prods the group into action or decision
11. Procedural technician - expedites group's movement by doing things for the group such as distributing materials, arranging seating
12. Recorder - writes down suggestions and group decisions, acts as the "group memory"

Group Building and Maintenance Roles

These are supportive roles which keep the group functioning together. There are seven:

1. Encourager - praises, agrees with and accepts the contributions of others
2. Harmonizer - mediates the differences between other members
3. Compromiser - modifies his own position in the interest of group harmony
4. Gate-keeper and expediter - keeps communication channels open by regulating its flow, and facilitating participation of others
5. Standard setter - expresses ideal standards for the group to aspire to
6. Group observer and commentator - comments on and interprets the process of the group
7. Follower - passively accepts ideas of others and goes along with the movement of the group

Individual Roles

These are opposed to group roles and indicate the use of the group to serve one's individual needs. These roles tend to interfere with group functioning. Benne and Sheats suggest that a high incidence of individual behaviors is symptomatic of various group malfunctions such as: inadequate group skills of members (including the leader), low level of group maturity, discipline and morale, or an inappropriately chosen and inadequately defined group task. There are eight individual roles defined by these authors:

1. Aggressor - deflates the status of others, expresses disapproval of the values, acts or feelings of others, attacks the group or group task, etc.
2. Blocker - tends to be negativistic or stubbornly resistant, opposing beyond reason or maintaining issues the group has rejected
3. Recognition-seeker - calls attention to self through boasting, acting in unusual ways or struggling to remain in the limelight.
4. Self-confessor - uses group as an audience for expressing non-group oriented feelings, insights or ideologies
5. Playboy - displays lack of involvement through joking, cynicism or nonchalance.

6. Dominator - monopolizes group through manipulation, flattery, giving directions authoritatively or interrupting the contributions of others
7. Help-seeker - looks for sympathy from the group through unreasonable insecurity, personal confusion or self-depreciation.
8. Special interest pleader - cloaks his or her own biases in the stereotypes of social causes, such as the laborer, the housewife, the homeless, or the small businessman.

Admittedly, the group roles are, in part, a function of the group's stage of development. More of the task and maintenance roles can be observed in a mature group than one that is less mature. No statements are made as to the relative value of the various roles. It can be assumed that all roles are equally valuable and necessary to the group's positive outcome. Too many opinion givers and not enough compromisers are likely to create chaos rather than productivity. A well-functioning group needs a balance of roles, and this requires members to take on a mixture of roles which are compatible.

As a learning experience, it is helpful to analyze its member roles. This gives members some feedback about what roles they tend to take on in groups and how they are contributing to the group outcome. It is easiest to see roles in groups that require extensive interaction, problem-solving and decision-making.

Role Analysis Exercise

Directions: After your group ends, take a few minutes to identify what members played the various identified roles. Give an example of the behavior that supports your choices.

A. Task Roles

Role	Member name	Sample comment or behavior
1. Initiator-contributor		
2. Information seeker		
3. Information giver		
4. Opinion seeker		
5. Opinion giver		
6. Elaborator		
7. Coordinator		
8. Orienter		
9. Evaluator-critic		
10. Energizer		
11. Procedural technician		
12. Recorder		

B. Maintenance Roles

Role	Member name	Sample comment or behavior
1. Encourager		
2. Harmonizer		
3. Compromiser		

Role Analysis Exercise (continued)

Role	Member name	Sample comment or behavior
4. Gate-keeper		
5. Standard-setter		
6. Group observer		
7. Follower		

C. Individual Roles

Role	Member name	Sample comment or behavior
1. Aggressor		
2. Blocker		
3. Recognition seeker		
4. Self-confessor		
5. Playboy		
6. Dominator		
7. Help-seeker		
8. Special interest Pleader		

Remember, a single member can take on several roles. After everyone has written down their ideas, group members should compare notes and discuss their answers and the reasons for them. See if the group can reach a consensus about who played which roles.

For further self-awareness, the questions in the Self Role Analysis Worksheet can be answered concerning your own role in the group.

Self Role Analysis Worksheet

1. What role(s) did you see yourself playing in the group?

2. Were these the same or different from the role(s) others saw you playing?

3. How does your role in this group compare with the one you usually play in groups?

4. What other roles would you like to try?

5. What comments or behaviors can you use to help you take on a new role?

Since flexibility in roles is considered a sign of maturity, it may be set as a goal in groups to have each member try a few new roles over the course of group meetings.

Special Patient Problems

It is evident from our discussion of individual roles, that certain member behaviors can interfere with or severely constrict the functioning of groups. Knowledge of group dynamics also helps the leader know how to deal with special problems. For example, if the leader understands why the monopolist needs to monopolize and how his or her behavior effects the other group members, then the type of therapeutic intervention needed can be determined. Sometimes the problems that arise are best dealt with by the leader, while others are handled more effectively by the group itself.

Yalom (1985) points out that all patients are problems. Indeed, patients are often assigned to therapy groups for the purpose of attempting to change problem behaviors. The behaviors to be reviewed here are: monopolizing, attention-getting, silence and psychosis. It is very important for the occupational therapist leading groups to gain an understanding of each member's needs and develop skills in handling problem behaviors.

These members who display these problem behaviors are those who play the individual roles in groups, often blocking the group's progress and frustrating its members. Dealing effectively with these patients in the group involves several challenges for the therapist. First, the therapist should develop an understanding of the individual dynamics of the patient: *What does this patient really need?* Secondly, the therapist needs to develop strategies for preserving the integrity and cohesiveness of the group: *What does the group need?* How can the leader handle this patient so that the group can continue to function therapeutically? Ideally both the patient need and the group need can be satisfied. Realistically, it is not always possible for the leader to do both. If a choice is to be made, the group should be preserved first, even if that means an individual member must leave it. A good group therapist will never sacrifice the whole group for the sake of an individual member.

The Monopolist

Harry came into the group angry. He refused to listen to the purpose of the group or to participate in the activity. "I'm not going to draw like I'm in kindergarten. Excuse me, but you girls (occupational therapy student leaders) don't know anything about alcohol abuse. When I was in County Hospital, they had me doing paintings and sculptures, and what-all, and it never did anything for me..." Five other members listened to this outburst in silence. They had heard Harry's routine before.

How should the leaders handle Harry? First, lets ask the two key questions. What does Harry need? Perhaps he needs to control the group, to maintain the group's (or leader's) attention; or perhaps he needs to avoid his own hurtful issues. What do the members of the group need? Probably, they need to get Harry to "shut up." However, when a silent group allows a monopolist to control things, there is always an element of ambivalence. In some ways, Harry may be serving their needs as well, particularly if they, too, wish to avoid revealing hurtful issues or feelings.

In this example, Harry is playing the role of the aggressor, by devaluing both the task and the leaders of the group. The leaders, in this case, are more likely to stop Harry's tirade by appealing to the other group members. Ask them, "Why do you allow Harry to monopolize your group? Why are you silent?" The group might be encouraged to give Harry feedback by completing the sentence, "When you speak like that it makes me feel."

If the group is able to express its frustration with Harry, then Harry might be helped by learning to control the behaviors that elicit negative feelings from others.

The Silent Member

Silent patients occur frequently in occupational therapy groups. In active groups, silent members may go unnoticed for a session or two, but will eventually block the group's progress. Why? Because, as the group becomes aware of a member's silence, members begin to imagine what the silent member must be thinking. Soon resentment develops over the silent, passive member's "not pulling his/her weight," in the group. In truth, a silent member might feel inadequate, out of tune with the others, and fearful of self-disclosure. What the group wants most is for the silent member to talk, and to allay its fears about what he/she may be thinking. For example, in a group of students, Patty usually made two or three non-committal comments in each session, just enough to keep her from being noticed. Patty's greatest fear was becoming the center of attention. But as members got to know one another through mutual participation in group activities, it soon became clear that no one was getting to know Patty. Two group members finally confronted her angrily at the beginning of a group. Once begun, she continued speaking in a very pressured way, hard to interrupt: "I've been listening to you all discussing your life in the dorms and your problems with your boyfriends. But I'm a commuter. I leave right after class and go to my evening job and I don't get home until midnight. On weekends I help my handicapped mother with the housework and help her shop and pay her bills. I don't have time for a boyfriend and homework too. I can't think about having fun when I'm wondering how I'll manage paying next semester's tuition or how I'll get the money to fix my car. I have nothing in common with this group. I'm not resentful or angry and I learn a lot from listening. But don't ask me to join in when I have nothing say." After allowing the group to respond, the occupational therapist suggested that the group try to find things Patty and they had in common, rather than things that singled her out as being different. Patty was still quiet, and had a hard time feeling like part of the group. But after this "event," the group no longer regarded her as an impediment. They empathized with her and collaborated to help involve her as much as she could tolerate.

Attention-Getting Behaviors

There are various forms of attention-getting behavior. Most represent self-centered patterns of interaction which reflect low self-esteem and the need for external evidence of one's worth. The three types we will discuss are self-depreciation, complaining and narcissism or self-love.

The Self-Depreciator

The self-depreciator is the patient whose stories you hear over and over. She's always putting herself down, and seems unresponsive to overtures of acceptance from others. Janice loved to do activities, so she participated willingly in occupational therapy group. But whenever she finished a project, she talked on and on about all of its flaws and imperfections. The group used to argue with her and tell her how nice her project looked. But the routine was repeated too often, so they stopped responding to Janice at all. This "fed up" group behavior made Janice feel all the more rejected.

Getting the group to help Janice to see her self-defeating behavior was a key intervention here. Through group feedback, Janice learned how she made her expectation of rejection a self-fulfilling prophecy. The leader encouraged Janice to accept the group's support and stop devaluing herself before the group gave up on her.

The Complainer

The help-rejecting complainer, referred to by Yalom as the "HRC" (1985, 389), chronically rejects the very help he asks for from the group. Yalom explains this behavior as unresolved dependency: the HRC is dependent on authoritative others, but at the same time, is unable to trust others. After the fifth or sixth "yes, but..." response, the group usually becomes frustrated and angry at having all it's advice rejected. The HRC is seen as using up a lot of time and energy and getting nowhere. Marge, for example, had chronic headaches and was addicted to several medications, which in turn, caused a barrage of other symptoms from constipation to irrational anger. An unknowing doctor tried to help Marge by lowering her pain medication prescription. Predictably, the doctor's well-meaning action not only did not help Marge, it made him the target of all her irrational anger. She complained incessantly in group and would not be consoled. Marge had once again painted herself into a corner. Not only had the group rejected her, but she had rejected the only one (the doctor) who had the credentials to help her with her addiction problem. Why does this happen? Because the patient is stuck in a self-defeating cycle (Figure 2-4).

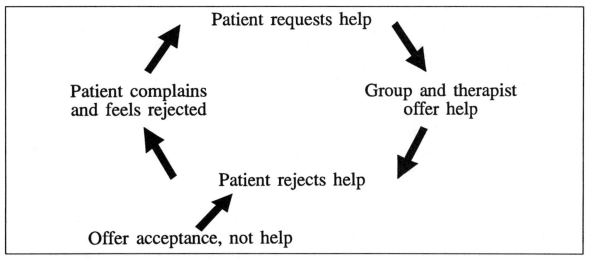

Figure 2-4. Self-defeating cycle of the HRC.

What to do? *Don't* give the patient the help requested. Why? Because she will reject the help and therefore reinforce the self-defeating cycle. The only hope for the HRC is to break the cycle. The therapist can help the group to empathize with Marge, to understand and acknowledge her feelings of defeat and frustration. As a bond with the group forms, the patient might be helped to see how her own behavior invites rejection.

The Narcissistic Member

These attention-seekers seem to demand the constant and undivided attention of the group. I've known doctors to come across this way in team meetings. Narcissistic patients have an exaggerated self-love; they feel they deserve concern, complements, gifts and surprises, although they give none of these to others. For example, Franklin, a small, clever and attractive man, seemed to have a natural talent for comedy. He held the group's attention with his humor, but rarely listened to the other members. Franklin did a lot of talking about the women he had affairs with; he couldn't understand why these relationships never lasted. The group's need was to have Franklin contribute to the group by listening to and empathizing with others.

Groups can be very useful to patients like this, who need to alter their perception of themselves and others. It is important, however, for the therapist to protect them because of their high degree of vulnerability. The group's feedback can be accepted if it is presented in a gentle and caring way. Franklin, for all his humorous over-confidence about his sex-appeal to women, had a very fragile sense of self-worth. He was highly dependent on the acceptance or rejection of others. The group, in their anger, could easily burst his bubble and their rejection would sink him to the depths of depression. Franklin needed the group's high regard to sustain him through their feedback about how his lack of caring makes them feel. The therapist might look for an opportunity to ask the group to comment about Franklin's rejection of them in ways that are not likely to evoke defensiveness.

Psychotic Patient Behavior

The patient who becomes psychotic and is out of touch with reality does not benefit from group treatment, according to Yalom. Irrational and illogical patients take up vast amounts of group energy, and may bring the group process to a halt. Such patients should be removed from the group until their psychosis comes under control through medical treatment. Posthuma, however, suggests that psychotic patients may benefit from occupational therapy group treatment in which the activity is the focus, rather than discussion and social interaction (Postuma 1989).

Additionally, psychosis may not always be easy to identify. Some patients continue to interact in a seemingly rational manner, and may deceive the group by creating distractions or personal crises to cover their breaks with reality. Patients with borderline personality disorder provide good examples of this problem behavior. Borderline patients have been identified as exceedingly difficult to treat. Yalom describes them as having an "outward veneer of integration" which "conceals a chaotic, primitive personality structure" (Yalom 1985, 407). Borderline patients often thrive in occupational therapy groups because they have developed a great deal of skill. Often they are excellent artists, craftsmen and writers, as well as convincing talkers. In groups, (as in life), they seem to go from crisis to crisis. Self-destructive acts can be an everyday occurrence, although often unpredictable. Group members and therapists alike are taken in by the borderline patient's great potential to achieve, and disappointed again and again by his impulsive self-destructiveness.

Group treatment can be valuable to the borderline patient, because of the many opportunities to test reality. Feedback from the group can keep his numerous perceptual distortions and primitive needs and fears in check. However, the therapist needs to be constantly in touch with the amount of the group's time and energy taken in meeting the needs of the borderline patient. Sometimes these patients leave little time for the other group members.

Termination of Groups

Finally, as the time for ending a group approaches, the leader will need to help the group through the process of termination. Some groups prepare for termination from the day they begin, while others avoid dealing with issues of termination altogether. The therapeutic learning that takes place in the group can be greatly enhanced by a good termination, or it can be destroyed by an inadequate termination. The leader should be keenly aware of the issues groups need to deal with in terminating so that she can help the group face them in a healthy and effective way.

This rather gruesome word *termination* is used here simply to mean the end of something. In the case of groups, it refers to the point at which groups cease to meet together as a group. Whether or not members expect to encounter one another as individuals in another context, termination of a group usually means the end of relationships as they exist within the group. The end of a group is a real loss, and involves some of the same feelings associated with other losses.

Termination, when faced directly, usually involves pain and anxiety. Group members tend to avoid these feelings in a number of ways: withdrawal, devaluing the importance of the group, anger toward the leader or other members, silence and inactivity or leaving the group prematurely. It was mentioned in the section on group development, that some research shows group regression as the end approaches. A group which has reached maturity may go backwards and re-enter a state of conflict prior to termination. Some groups just ignore the impending termination by bringing up new issues as if the group would continue as usual.

A healthy termination is never easy. However, leaders can help group members to go through the process, which involves several steps.

1. Review the group experience, the goals, and the learning that took place over the life of the group. Even though members may wish to devalue the group, the leader can encourage members to verbalize the goals they have accomplished, or can help them recall positive learning experiences.
2. Review concerns and feelings regarding separation and loss. A good therapist will encourage the expression of painful, sad, angry or anxious feelings to prepare the members for separation. Often the leader will experience these feelings and can share them with the group as an example.
3. Use counselling skills. Empathy and confrontation (detailed in chapter 3) are often useful in this process to help members acknowledge their feelings instead of avoiding them.
4. Finish unfinished business. This seems obvious, but there may be various reasons why members wish to avoid doing it. A therapist should encourage members to bring up issues that are pending, and follow up on past conflicts to bring closure.
5. Give feedback on skills learned. Group members may be engaged in giving one another feedback about changes they have made, or learning what has been gained from the group's activities.
6. Help generalize learning. As a way to help members accept separation, an emphasis can be placed on how what was learned in the group can be practiced and applied elsewhere. When members understand how they can apply their skills to their lives outside of the group, they can move on without diminishing the importance of their group experience.

Summary

Students learn best about group dynamics through experience. So it is recommended that students meet in a series of six to ten group sessions. These can be led by peers, or can follow the format of Chapter 10, led by an instructor.

As a way to enhance an awareness of group dynamics, it is suggested that the following outline be used to record student reactions after each group session.

Personal Group Reaction Outline

Title _____ Date of session _____
(a few words expressing theme)

Seating Pattern Diagram
1. Draw a diagram of the seating arrangement, listing names of each member present and his or her position within the group.
2. Discuss significance of seating pattern, positions near leader, opposite leader, pairing, subgroups.
3. Note absences and impact of these.

Norms: Identify "rules" of the group (confidentiality, respect, etc.). What behaviors are acceptable to the group? Not acceptable? Each week note any changes in group norms from previous weeks.

Content: Identify the major discussion topics of the group.

Process:
1. Theme - Based on the topics discussed, identify the predominant theme of the session in a few words or a phrase (this becomes the "title" of your paper). The theme should have both a content and a process (or feeling) component. Then explain how you arrived at this theme. How do the topics reflect the theme and why were they verbalized (or not verbalized) in this manner?
2. Stage - Identify the stage of development you think your group is in and why.
3. Verbal Communication - What significant interpersonal interactions took place between group members? Be sure to name names. Vagueness is not helpful to the understanding of process. Interpret what was implied or hidden in the group discussion. What subjects were avoided and why?
4. Non-Verbal Communication - What was the general mood of the group? What was communicated by non-verbal behaviors of members, especially feelings of members? Interpret significance. How did non-verbal behaviors affect group functioning?

Personal Reaction: Identify your role and impact you had on the group. Describe your personal feelings.
1. How did you respond to this group?
2. How do you feel about your relationship to the group?
3. How did you react to the leadership style?

Self Evaluation: What did you learn about yourself today in group? (Strengths, weaknesses, values, interactive style).

Goal: What are your personal goals for the next session?

Bibliography

Benne K. and Sheats P. Functional roles of group members. *J of Social Issues* 2(4)123-135, 1948.

Bion W. *Experiences in Groups and Other Papers*. NY: Basic Books, 1961.

Cathcart R. and Samovar L. *Small Group Communication, A Reader*. 2nd ed. Dubuque, Iowa: W.C.Brown Co, 1974.

Corey G, Corey MS, Callanan P, Russel J. *Group Techniques*. rev. ed. Pacific Grove, CA: Brooks/Cole, 1988.

Egan G. *The Skilled Helper*. Monterey CA: Brooks/Cole, 1986.

Hare A. *Handbook of Small Group Research*. 2nd ed. NY: Macmillan, 1976.

Posthuma B. *Small Groups in Therapy Settings: Process and Leadership*. Boston: Little Brown, 1989.

Schutz W. The interpersonal underworld. *Harvard Business Review*, 36(4) 123-135, 1958.

Tuckman B. Developmental sequence in small groups. *Psychological Bulletin*, 63(6) 384-399, 1965.

Yalom I. *The Theory and Practice of Group Psychotherapy*. 3rd ed. NY: Basic Books, 1985.

Yalom I. *Inpatient Group Psychotherapy*. NY: Basic Books, 1983.

SECTION TWO

Group Guidelines from Seven Frames of Reference

Introduction

Yalom (1985) writes that although there are presently many diverse "group therapies," there is a body of research that has been derived from a common ancestor. The oldest and most researched group is the long term outpatient therapy group. This group consists of the most highly motivated patients and the most ambitious goals: to offer symptomatic relief and also to change character structure.

Once the basic dynamics and principles of this higher level group are mastered, (as in Chapters 1 and 2) the student can then modify these to fit many specific clinical situations. Yalom suggests three steps for doing this: assessment of the clinical situation, formulation of goals and modification of technique. I have adopted Yalom's sound judgment in using these steps to plan occupational therapy groups, but have added an additional important step: identification and application of a frame of reference.

Regarding the position of frames of reference in practice, Mosey writes that "many authors ... (have) recognize(d) that no theory can be directly applied. A theory must first be transformed through a linking structure into usable information" (Mosey 1989, 195). Mosey suggests that our research should focus on the development, refinement and evaluation of the effectiveness of frames of reference.

Occupational therapy uses a method called "extrapolation" (Mosey 1989, 197) to make theory usable, involving several steps as follows:

1) identification of appropriate theories
2) selection of useful concepts and postulates
3) combining concepts and postulates from various compatible theories and
4) reformulating of the selected concepts and postulates to provide guidelines for treatment.

In addressing the problem of planning and leading occupational therapy groups, I have used a similar technique in applying theory.

Identification of Appropriate Theories

First, I have identified seven appropriate practice theories: humanistic, psychoanalytic, cognitive, developmental, neurodevelopmental, the model of human occupation and acquisitional. Some leaders in our profession would take exception to my choice of frames of reference. The psychoanalytic, humanistic and developmental chapters draw widely upon psychological theory. The acquisitional and neurodevelopmental chapters draw mainly from the fields of neurology, anatomy and physiology (and related medical fields). The model of human occupation, while identified by most as original to occupational therapy, draws upon systems theory which is used widely in business and was originally derived from physics. My point is, most of the theoretical concepts that make up occupational therapy frames of reference have also been researched and applied in other disciplines. What makes these frames of reference different from similar theories in psychology and medicine is that the concepts were reorganized in a way that can guide us in planning and leading occupational therapy groups.

Selecting Useful Concepts and Postulates

In describing each frame of reference, compatible concepts which are applicable to occupational therapy group treatment are selected from various theories. First, each concept or basic assumption is described according to the source or author where it originated. Then the relationship of the concepts to occupational therapy groups is facilitated through examples and learning exercises.

Combining Concepts and Postulates

Compatible concepts are combined from various theories to formulate a point of view on function, dysfunction, change and motivation. A frame of reference should guide our understanding of illness and disability in our patients. Before jumping into group treatment, occupational therapists should have some understanding of the state of health of the group members, and this understanding is different in each frame of reference. The definition of dysfunction can range from neurological malfunctioning in the neurodevelopmental frame of reference, to the presence of unconscious conflicts in the psychoanalytic frame, to the lack of adaptive skill development in the acquisitional frame. Principles or postulates regarding change (Mosey 1981) are the assumptions derived from theory that help us formulate how treatment will work. These are the "principles by which prevention of dysfunction occurs, function is maintained, interfering behavior is managed and an individual is assisted in moving from a state of dysfunction to a state of function"(Mosey 1981, 141).

Mosey further suggests that principles of intervention begin with the function to be developed (e.g. trunk balance, self-esteem), and end with the nature of the external environment that is likely to enact this therapeutic change. In other words, these principles help us predict how change will occur, and guide our designing of occupational therapy activities that will facilitate the development of function. For example, in using a developmental frame of reference for a group of elderly Parkinson's patients, the postulate regarding intervention may be as follows: a sense of integrity and acceptance of one's life and death may be facilitated by participation in group activities where past accomplishments are the focus. In an acquisitional frame of reference for the same patients, the postulate regarding change might be socially acceptable eating habits may be learned through the use of weighted utensils combined with peer examples. Each of these frames of reference suggests a different definition of function and dysfunction, different goals to be addressed, and a different kind of activity. Thus, the important parts of occupational therapy group treatment are addressed in the different frames. Within each chapter on frame of reference, concepts are applied to group structure, limitations, role of the leader, appropriate goals and suggested activities as examples.

Reformulating Concepts to Provide Guidelines for Treatment

To provide the student with a concrete idea of how groups should be run in each of the frames of reference, the seven step format for group leadership described in Chapter 1 is modified for each frame of reference covered. The introduction, use of activity, sharing, generalizing and application are summarized with suggested modifications based on the concepts of each frame of reference. It is hoped that with this breakdown, the application of theory will be, at least partly, demystified.

Bibliography

Llorens L & Gillette N. Nationally speaking -- The challenge for research in a practice profession. *AJOT*, 39,143-145, 1985.

Mosey A. *Occupational Therapy: Configuration of a Profession*. NY: Raven, 1981.

Mosey A. The proper focus of scientific inquiry in occupational therapy: Frames of reference. *OTJR*: 9, 4, 195-201, 1989.

Yalom I. *The Theory and Practice of Group Psychotherapy*. NY: Basic Books, 1985.

Chapter

3

An Existential/Humanistic Approach

The existential/humanistic frame of reference seems to correspond closely to what we have come to know as group dynamics theory. Many of the general concepts reviewed in Chapter 2 seem to rely on the basic assumptions from existential and humanistic psychotherapy. The humanistic approach is also a major contributor to the core philosophy of occupational therapy. As the basic assumptions of existential and humanistic theory are reviewed, this connection will become evident.

The humanistic philosophy focuses on mankind as separate from animals and attempts to define those characteristics which are uniquely human. The value of human beings is paramount in the humanistic view. People are seen as equally valuable, regardless of their race, religion, sex, level of intellectual ability, socioeconomic position or state of health.

The very roots of occupational therapy, back at the turn of the century, reflect these humanistic beliefs. The "philosophical base of occupational therapy," adopted by the American Occupational Therapy Association (AOTA) in April 1979, states that "human beings are able to influence their physical and mental health and their social and physical environment through purposeful activity" and "adaptation is a change in function that promotes survival and self-actualization" (Hopkins and Smith 1983, 27). The Principles of Occupational Therapy Ethics of the AOTA continue to emphasize the rights of all human beings to equal treatment and to advocate the rights of the handicapped.

However, as Mosey (1981) reminds us, a philosophy (fundamental belief) or a theory (concepts and postulates), cannot be directly applied. So, after reviewing the basic assumptions of existentialist and humanistic theory, the applications (plans of action) described by Carl Rogers and Gerard Egan will be discussed. These authors/therapists present applications of humanistic theory which are particularly useful to occupational therapists. Their techniques can be identified as helping guide our interventions in occupational therapy groups, as well as our choice of activities.

Basic Assumptions

Existential Concepts

Existential theory can be seen as the forerunner of humanism. The major contributions of the existentialists lie in two key concepts: freedom and anxiety.

Freedom

Freedom implies that an individual has a capacity for self-awareness and awareness of his environment that allows him to make choices. An individual who is aware, need not allow his present behavior to be determined by others, his situation or his past experiences. He alone is responsible for his own life dilemmas. Therapy that utilizes this approach is aimed at getting patients to see that they have choices, have always had choices, and helps them take responsibility for the choices that have made them who they are now. Adults can stop blaming their parents for their shortcomings, and instead, take on the responsibility of correcting them. The concept of freedom to choose is what allows patients to take charge of their own lives, to leave the past behind and to make positive changes for the future.

Anxiety

Anxiety, in the existentialist view, is a necessary condition of living. Rollo May defines anxiety as "the threat to our existence or to values we identify with our existence" (1977, 205). The concept is based on the idea that our existence or "being" (May and Yalom 1989) has no intrinsic predetermined meaning. The meaning of life is developed by each individual for himself. Thus in therapy, there is an emphasis on one's individual values, and in finding or defining what activities are meaningful to the individual. It is the existentialist view that while too much anxiety can immobilize a person, a certain amount of anxiety is normal and positive. It is anxiety that alerts one that all is not well, and that a change is needed. In this case, anxiety is seen as a motivator to make necessary changes in behavior, values or life structure in order to maintain or promote healthy functioning.

Humanistic Concepts

The humanistic approach is overwhelmingly positive and is appealing to most therapists. Carl Rogers was perhaps its major spokesman. Rogers developed what is known as nondirective counseling, based on the assumption that the patient really knows what is best for him. Rogers viewed his patients with "unconditional positive regard" and allowed them to choose the direction of therapy, to set their own goals and to provide their own solutions to problems (Rogers 1967). Abraham Maslow added significantly to humanistic thinking also. The key concepts of his humanistic approach are: respect, genuineness, non-judgmental acceptance, deep understanding and self-actualization.

Respect

Respect in therapy is not a technique, but an attitude toward the patient. In the humanistic approach, the therapist sees the patient as the only real expert on his own life. Therefore, the therapist makes no predetermined assumptions about the patient, but seeks to learn all about him by asking open ended questions and getting him to talk about himself as much as possible. Yalom translates this idea in his approach to group treatment, by encouraging group members to respect each other and to talk to each other as much as possible. Respect also includes a belief that when people are realistically aware of their problems, they are capable of creating their own solutions. Therefore, suggestions and advice-giving are discouraged, and replaced by responses that show empathy. Empathy is expressed by both therapist and group members by statements that not only reflect what the patient has said, but also acknowledge how the patient is feeling. For example, a patient presents the problem that his wife doesn't understand his need to grieve the death of his mother. The therapist would encourage the group to ask for appropriate details in order to gain a thorough understanding of how this patient feels. Then empathy would be expressed with a statement like "You must be feeling abandoned when your wife cannot share your grief about the loss of your mother." Statements such as this encourage the patient to trust the therapist and/or group members and to move ahead to even greater self-disclosure.

Genuineness

Genuineness is also an attitude rather than a technique. It means that the therapist expresses real emotional responses to the patient. Patients are keen observers and are quick to sense any dishonesty on the part of therapists. When the therapist tries to cover up anger or frustation, the patient usually senses something wrong and the effect is often silence and withdrawal of trust. It is only by expressing negative feelings that honest communication with the patient is facilitated. This is not to suggest that the therapists' anger (or other feelings) should be expressed indiscriminately. On the contrary, it takes considerable skill and self-understanding for a therapist to express feelings in a way that is therapeutic (Egan 1986).

The value of genuineness has a profound effect upon groups. When the therapist encourages the members to be genuine, the responses they give to one another are much more meaningful and helpful. In the initial stages of groups, it is a natural tendency for members to hold back in their responses to one another. Patients are often reluctant to express negative feelings toward other members. Reasons for this have been discussed in the chapter on group dynamics. After members have established a certain degree of trust in one another, they feel much more inclined to share their real feelings. It is one of the therapist's roles to establish an atmosphere of safety and trust which allows group members to be genuine in their responses to one another.

Non-Judgmental Acceptance

Non-judgmental acceptance refers to the therapist's relationship with the patient as one of caring. In the humanistic approach, the patient is accepted for the human being that he is, regardless of his feelings or his behavior. This "unconditional positive regard" allows the patient to reveal all his inner feelings and secrets without fearing the therapist's rejection. According to Rogers, research indicates that "the greater the degree of caring, prizing, accepting and valuing the client in a non-possessive way, the greater the chance that therapy will be successful" (Corey 1991, 214). The humanistic therapist needs to be very careful not to allow his own values to enter into the therapeutic relationship. Judgments of bad and good feelings or bad and good behavior have no place in the humanistic approach.

Being judged by others is one of the greatest fears patients have in the group setting. For example, when a patient speaks in the group, he is often uncomfortable with the silence of others. Patients often imagine that silent members are secretly disapproving of what is being said. It is most important for the therapist to establish the norm or expectation early in the group that members not judge one another in this way. All members have a right to have feelings and feelings are neither good nor bad. Likewise, behavior should not be judged for itself, but looked upon in the context of the individual's perceptions of self and environment. If a patient got drunk on a weekend pass, this behavior can be seen as one of several responses the patient could have to a stressful situation. The object is not to condemn the behavior but to understand it and examine its effect on the patient.

Deep Understanding

In the humanistic approach, behavior change is considered to be the by-product of a deep self-understanding. For this reason, considerable time and energy in therapy is devoted to uncovering hidden aspects of the self. In occupational therapy groups, structured activities are often helpful in fostering self-understanding among group members. The therapist should continue to gather information from the patients until she can almost see the world through the patient's eyes. Only then is the therapist able to assist the patient in changing his behavior. New therapists have a tendency to push for behavior change too quickly. In their desire to be helpful, new therapists might even make a suggestion in the form of a question, i.e., "Have you tried talking to your wife instead of just getting drunk?" Such a question reveals a lack of respect as well as understanding. Questions should focus on further defining the problem until it is thoroughly explored. When it is revealed that the patient depends on his wife so much that he cannot risk disagreeing with her, then getting drunk to numb the pain is less contemptible. Furthermore, the problem is redefined not as one of drunkenness, but one of dependency. That dependency may be further explained by a lack of trust in oneself. Problems are seldom as simple as they may seem. Rogers believes that "when therapists can grasp the present experience of the client's private world as the client sees and feels it without losing the separateness of their own identity, then constructive change is likely to occur" (Corey 1991, 214).

Self-Actualization

Self-actualization is the innate tendency of all human beings to achieve their potential. This concept assumes that each of us has within us an inherent potential that we can actualize and through which we can find meaning. Maslow, the chief proponent of this concept, places self-actualization at the top of a continuum called the hierarchy of needs. Maslow sees at the core of human nature a push to satisfy the needs which ensure physical and psychological survival. The satisfaction of each need is a necessary prerequisite to the search for satisfaction of the next. Thus, in Maslow's hierarchy: 1) physiological needs, 2) safety needs, 3) needs for belonging and love and 4) esteem needs are all prerequisites to the need for self-actualization. In his book *Toward a Psychology of Being*, Maslow elaborates the idea of self-actualization in his discussion of "peak experiences." These experiences are difficult to describe, but widely documented, according to Maslow. They are moments of ecstasy, of self-discovery and brilliant creativity or vision; moments when suddenly one's views of himself and the world change permanently—forever. Peak experiences are said to cause symptoms to disappear; they can change self-perception in a healthy direction and can release the person for greater creativity, expressiveness and growth. "The person, (after such experiences), is more apt to feel that life in general is worthwhile, even if it is usually drab, pedestrian, painful or ungratifying, since beauty, excitement, honesty, play, goodness, truth and meaningfulness have been demonstrated to him to exist" (Maslow 1968, 101).

If only we, as therapists, could make our patients feel that life is worthwhile in this way!

The humanistic view of the world seems so optimistic, so holistic, so simple. Now let us apply some of its ideas to our view of patients.

Function and Dysfunction

In the humanistic view, a healthy functioning individual is one who is self-actualized, who is functioning close to his potential. Such a person is aware of the freedom to make choices, and takes responsibility for the decisions of the past. He or she is not inhibited by guilt over lost opportunities, and does not blame others for his or her dilemmas. A healthy person works toward satisfying his or her own physiological and psychological needs, and chooses an environment and life structure that allows growth and expression. Anxiety is replaced by meaningfulness and purpose; the individual feels good about him or herself.

Dysfunction would be the opposite of all these. But there is the difficulty. We as therapists need to find out where the dysfunction lies—where our patient is stuck, and the obstacles preventing him or her from pursuing self-actualization. Perhaps the patient is not aware of the freedom to make choices. Many patients I have worked with have felt so defeated by the "system," by the bureaucracy of governments and organizations or by the prejudices of society, that they no longer exercise their ability to choose. Many have had negative life experiences rather than "peak" experiences. Perhaps their more basic needs are not being satisfied, they feel unsafe, unloved or like they don't belong. People with handicaps, both mental and physical, often feel they are misfits, controlled by others, victims of circumstance, incapacitated by anxiety and prevented from enjoying the fulfillments of life that "normal" people enjoy. As therapists, we may need to listen to and endure with our patients a great deal of pain before we can help them begin to find the more positive aspects of themselves.

Change and Motivation

Humanists and existentialists often address motivation in their writings. Maslow views need satisfaction as a kind of thrust for survival. But this changes from physiological survival to psychological survival as it approaches the top of the needs hierarchy. Self-actualization is seen not as a search for what is missing, but an innate drive toward self-fulfillment. This differs somewhat from the existentialist view that anxiety is the major motivator, that the search for structure and meaning is largely motivated by the desire to escape the anxiety of meaninglessness and nothingness. In humanistic theory, there is an assumption that people have a natural tendency to improve the quality of their lives. This idea is certainly compatible with the basic tenets of occupational therapy. Perhaps we would add that our plan of action to improve the quality of life is the engagement in meaningful occupation.

Of central concern in the health professions is the knowledge of how change occurs, since it is upon this knowledge that we base our treatment. Here again, psychological theorists give us many clues. The humanists say that we cannot change our patients, that they must desire to change themselves. The function of the therapist is to create an atmosphere of safety and to help the patient build the kind of self-image and self-understanding that increases the likelihood of positive change. The humanistic therapist does this through the therapeutic relationship and through the facilitation of therapeutic groups. Rogers said that behavior change is really a by-product of a deep self-understanding. To change their lives in a positive way, patients must first feel and believe that they have the strength and the power to make changes. This requires a feeling of self-worth and self-esteem as well as a belief that one has the needed skills and capacities required. A prerequisite for change is the belief that change is possible. All of these are appropriate issues to be addressed in occupational therapy groups.

Group Treatment

Yalom in his *Theory and Practice of Group Psychotherapy* (1985) describes a basically existential humanistic approach. Patients are treated in groups not only because it is practical, but because of the many unique advantages that only a group can offer in treatment. The goals for an individual in this frame of reference have mostly to do with increasing self-understanding, self-worth and self-actualization. In the group setting, members are expected to discuss their own lives, their problems and successes. Through their self-disclosure, members develop relationships with one another and learn to trust one another. The feedback and support they give one another is of far greater value than what they can get from any individual.

Furthermore, many of the therapeutic factors described by Yalom (instillation of hope, universality, altruism, group cohesiveness and interpersonal learning) will help the members achieve their goals. The therapeutic factors are those aspects of groups which make them therapeutic. Instillation of hope conveys the positive expectation members have at the outset of groups that the group experience will help them. Patients in group treatment often feel great relief when they discover that their problems are not unique, that others share their misery (universality). Altruism implies that patients benefit not only by receiving from others, but also from giving. Learning to give to others in the group may in fact be the most important lesson of all. Group cohesiveness has been described as the final and most desirable stage of group development. It is an attraction for each other that is shared by all its members. Cohesiveness makes posssible all the positive, productive work that can be accomplished by the mature group described in Chapter 2. Interpersonal learning incorporates a broad range of factors about the give and take of emotional and social relationships to one another. The reader is referred to Yalom (1985), Chapters 1 and 2, for further discussion of the therapeutic factors of groups.

A humanistic group is best suited to a higher functioning clientele. It is the approach suggested for personal/professional growth of student groups or staff groups. A certain level of self-awareness is expected, and members should be able to communicate their self-perceptions to the group reasonably well. In short, members must be capable of **insight**. Insight means not only acknowledging one's own problematic behavior but having some understanding of the reasons behind it.

For example, I have treated groups of substance abuse patients using this approach. Most of these patients have been employed, and have developed intimate relationships with others, and have in times past functioned in the world with relative success. Self-awareness activities and discussion of values are helpful in defining problems. These patients understood all too well how abusing substances interfered with functioning, since many had endured severe losses—spouses, jobs, financial losses—due to their drug/alcohol habits. They were able to discuss the dilemmas and the pain openly and to help each other learn alternative strategies. Often their problems seemed to be related to an inability to assert themselves emotionally or to cope with stress. There are other problems, of course, but occupational therapy groups in this example tended to focus on issues of assertiveness and stress management.

Role of the Leader

The occupational therapist who follows a humanistic frame of reference focuses on skills which help develop the therapeutic relationship. These skills will be used extensively in planning and leading occupational therapy groups. A thorough knowledge of group dynamics is extremely important in helping him to select members, set goals and plan appropriate activities.

A democratic leadership style (facilitator, advisor) is the most appropriate for humanistic groups. This gives group members an active part in the direction and process of therapy, while allowing the leader to guide them through the establishment of therapeutic norms.

Knowledge of the stages of groups is important, as well as what skills are appropriate for each stage. The reader is referred to Gerard Egan's *The Skilled Helper* (1986) for a more thorough discussion of these skills. Egan's text is intended for teaching basic counseling skills for those who will be doing individual psychotherapy. However, the stages of counseling which parallel the development of groups and the use of specific skills in group intervention will be the emphasis here.

Egan describes three stages of counselling: I - Problem Definition, II - Self Understanding and III - Behavior Change. Stage I is concerned with problem definition. This stage is parallel to the beginning stage of a group, in which members get to know one another and begin to lay the ground rules for how they will interact. The skills Egan suggests for this stage are attending, concreteness and primary accurate empathy.

Attending

Attending is something most of us do without even thinking about it. The leader of the group needs to be especially alert and observant since she is attending to not one, but several people at one time. Attending refers to the attentive physical presence the therapist focuses on the patient. It is evident even before anyone begins to speak. Taking note of appearance, body language, posture, seating position, eye contact and facial expression are all part of attending. The therapist gets from these factors important clues as to how members are feeling and how the group is likely to respond to various activities or interventions.

Skill Practice in Attending

To help you become aware of how powerful these first impressions really are, try sitting in a group for the first few minutes without speaking and do the following:
1. Draw a diagram of where people are seated in the room
2. Write a one or two word phrase describing the appearance of each member. For example:
    Glenn - sloppy, poor hygiene
    Mary - dressed up, neat
    Sue - provocative, overly made up
    Joe - preppie, well-groomed

71

3. Write one or two adjectives to describe the posture of each member. For example:
   Glenn - relaxed, slouching
   Mary - watchful, tense
   Sue - uncomfortable, fidgety
   Joe - alert, open
4. Note with whom each member has eye contact. For example:
   Glenn - looks at no one, looks down
   Mary - looks at everyone
   Sue - looks only at Joe
   Joe - looks at leader primarily
5. Write a word of feeling describing the emotional message given by the facial expression of each. For example:
   Glenn - defiant
   Mary - anxious, fearful
   Sue - distracted, blunted
   Joe - eager, anticipating

It is most helpful to put the descriptions of each individual together so you can begin to get a more complete picture of each (First Impressions Worksheet).

Knowing these impressions before starting the group, the leader can predict some responses that can be expected from the four patients. Even if the therapist doesn't know anything about the patients except their names and ages, an observant leader will begin to adapt his or her approach to the group to accommodate the different expectations.

Which of these patients is most likely to be cooperative? Uncooperative? Which patient is most likely to disrupt the group? Which member might be expected to leave prematurely? Attending and forming impressions of members becomes second nature to the skilled therapist, but the beginning therapist perhaps needs some practice. The following exercise may be used to practice these observations on your own group.

First Impressions Worksheet

Practice Skill in Attending: List names of group members in first column. Then use one or two descriptive words to denote appearance, posture and facial expression. Before beginning to speak, note the persons each member makes eye contact with. This information will make up your first impressions of group members.

Member name	Appearance	Posture	Eye contact	Facial expression
1.				
2.				
3.				
4.				
5.				
6.				
7.				
8.				

Concreteness

Concreteness refers to the ability to elicit specific information about a patient/problem. If the humanistic therapist's goal is to obtain a thorough understanding of the patient, many clarifying questions must ultimately be asked. The most basic skill in concreteness is to ask open-ended questions. These are questions that cannot be answered with a simple "yes" or "no." Open-ended questions encourage the patient to clarify his perceptions, elaborate on important points and give specific personal examples. A therapist may use open questions to get the patient to discover concrete solutions to problems, but that often happens in a later stage of treatment.

Constructing open-ended questions is not always as easy as it seems. Some beginning therapists are in the bad habit of asking closed questions one after the other, and this kind of habit is hard to break. Consider the following opening of an occupational therapy session:

OT:	Would you like to do some drawing today?
Joe:	No.
OT:	Are you too tired?
Joe:	Yes.
OT:	Can you just talk to me for a while?
Joe:	I'd rather not.
OT:	Do you find it hard to talk?
Joe:	Yes.
OT:	Why?
Joe:	I don't know.

Now consider the following alternative opening:

OT:	To begin our session, I'd like to learn how well you express your feelings. What can you tell me about how you're feeling right now?
Joe:	Nothing.
OT:	What makes it difficult to talk about feelings with me?
Joe:	It's nothing against you, I'm just in a bad mood.
OT:	What put you in a bad mood?
Joe:	My doctor just told me I can't go home this weekend.

In leading occupational therapy groups, open questions are more effective because they encourage communication and interaction among members. Closed questions tend to cut off communication. This is an important point to remember when planning questions for discussion when processing an activity group. In asking open questions, it seems most useful to begin with the words "what" or "how." Using the word "why" is not advisable because it tends to elicit vague answers, and because it may sound judgmental, reminding some patients of their angry parents' interrogations. Also, avoid beginning a question with "do you, can you, would you, are you" or "have you," because these can easily be answered with "yes" or "no," as observed in the above example.

Open-Ended Questions Worksheet

Directions: In each of the following examples, respond to the patient with an open question that can:

    a. elicit more specific information
    b. focus the discussion on a specific problem
    c. help define the problem

1. "I am always so unlucky!"
Response:

2. "No matter what I do, I can't win."
Response:

3. "I'm not thinking right today."
Response:

4. "Boy, did I have a boring weekend!"
Response:

5. "My doctor gave me new medication, and I'm just not myself."
Response:

6. "Life is so unfair. Do you think there's any justice in the world?"
Response:

7. "What good does it do to write down a schedule? When I go home, it's all for nothing."
Response:

8. "I'm really afraid to talk about how I feel."
Response:

9. "Just let well enough alone. I feel great today."
Response:

10. "Why should I care what my mother thinks?"
Response:

Primary Accurate Empathy

Primary accurate empathy is discussed by several humanistic theorists, particularly Carl Rogers. The importance of its use early in therapy cannot be overemphasized. Primary accurate empathy is the reflection of the feeling and content expressed by the patient. If composed and delivered effectively, an empathetic comment from either the therapist or another group member will convince the patient that he is being listened to and understood. The effect of empathy is to encourage this patient to open up even more. Primary accurate empathy, used often in groups, will help build an atmosphere of safety and trust, and will help the group progress toward a state of cohesiveness.

Primary accurate empathy is considered "primary" because it doesn't reach far below the surface. It reflects, but does not repeat, what the patient has actually said. Empathy requires that the feeling of the patient be recognized, and that may require careful observation of non-verbal cues as well as what the patient actually says. (In the practice exercise, you'll just have to read between the lines.) The "accurate" part of empathy requires that the emotion be identified accurately. Emotions vary in both kind and intensity. Some psychologists have divided feelings into the categories of sad, mad, bad (and) glad. It isn't enough to just say "you feel angry." Anger varies from low intensity, like *annoyed*, or *perturbed*, to very high intensity, like *rage*. Patients often do not have a very wide "feeling" vocabulary; many are not used to expressing their feelings in words. Often patients need the help of the therapist to find right words to describe their feelings accurately.

When practicing this skill, we will use a sentence completion to facilitate finding the right feeling words. We will complete the sentence, "You feel _____ because _____ ." "You feel" refers to the feeling word that best reflects how the patient is feeling. "Because" refers to the thoughts or behaviors that are seen to have caused the feeling. When leading a group, you'll learn to use your own words to show empathy. Now try the following exercise.

Primary Accurate Empathy Worksheet

Directions: After reading each patient's comment in group, write a response which completes the sentence: "You feel _____ because _____ ." and communicates:

a. What emotion that patient is feeling (as accurately as possible).

b. A summary of the thoughts or behaviors that are seen to have caused the feeling.

1. "I can't draw very well (shows a very faintly drawn picture to the group). This is supposed to be my sofa and my dog."
   You feel _____ because _____ .

2. "He just accused me of being prejudiced! I say he's a moron!"
   You feel _____ because _____ .

3. "Brian is doing so well. He's leaving tomorrow to start a new life, and here I am, still in the hospital."
   You feel _____ because _____ .

4. "Can I leave now? This group is making me very upset, especially when Mark sounds so angry."
   You feel _____ because _____ .

5. "This group just isn't helping me. None of you understand what I'm going through!"
   You feel _____ because _____ .

6. "I didn't want to come to occupational therapy group today. Setting goals is too much work."
   You feel _____ because _____ .

7. "When Laurie tells me I'm being insensitive, I don't know what she means."
   You feel _____ because _____ .

8. "All I know is that I'm restricted to the ward again. They seem to like punishing me."
   You feel _____ because _____ .

9. "My boyfriend always picks on me when he's had a bad day. Now I am too upset to participate in this group."
   You feel _____ because _____ .

10. Laurie (crying), "I don't know why I'm so upset. Just hearing Roy talk about being old and alone. He reminds me of my grandfather who died two months ago."
    You feel _____ because _____ .

According to Egan (1986), the goal of stage II in counseling is self-understanding. The middle stage of group development is more complex than this, with its sub-groups, leadership struggles and questioning of purpose/value, but the outcome is still a greater self-understanding. It is helpful to groups if the leader uses and teaches the skills of stage II to get through this vital phase of group development. The skills of stage II are immediacy, advanced accurate empathy and confrontation.

Immediacy

Immediacy is the direct mutual communication between therapist and patient. It enables the therapist to discuss openly and directly what is happening in the here and now of their interpersonal relationship. It is an invitation to process the relationship, and this is how it is best used in groups. When a group bogs down, and nothing seems to be happening, a question like: "What is happening right now?" or "What do you think the silence means?" will serve to refocus the group on its own process. The group's relationship to its leader is commonly a troubled one in stage 2, with which immediacy can help. For example, the leader can often sense anger, resentment or rebellion in the members and invite the group to discuss it. She could ask: "Are you angry with me for insisting that you give each other constructive feedback?" This direct question encourages the members to examine their own feelings about the leader, an essential task in the "control" stage of groups. Trust is another important issue to help therapist immediacy. A comment like "I can see that you're having a hard time trusting one another in this group today," will invite the group members to examine their relationships with one another.

Practice of Immediacy Worksheet

Directions: In the following examples, respond with a direct question or statement that encourages the group to examine its here and now relationships.

1. Group of adolescents hospitalized for drug abuse.

   Tina: "If we discuss our problems in group, you'll just tell our parents. They're the ones who sent us here in the first place."

   Bob: "Yeah, how do we know you won't rat on us?"

   Mikki: "I'm not telling you nothin'. I may have to come to this group, but I don't have to talk."

Therapist response:

2. Group of eating disorder patients, working on vocational readiness. This group has chosen to do one small craft project after another. None of the members have opted to take on anything more challenging; yet three of the members face discharge with only three or four more occupational therapy sessions.

Therapist response:

3. Group of arthritis patients attending the third session of a leisure planning group.

   Morgan: "What are we in this group for anyway? All I want to do is go back to work. Then I won't have any leisure time."

   Jackie: "I stopped participating in sports back in high school. Sure, it would be good for me, but it's just too much effort."

   Ellie: "Sure my doctor told me I need to plan time for relaxation and enjoyment, but I'm not sure I need someone telling me how or when to do it."

Therapist response:

Advanced Accurate Empathy

Advanced accurate empathy (AAE) goes a step further than primary accurate empathy. This skill enables the therapist to bring feelings and thoughts that the patient may only be implying to the forefront. Therapists find AAE difficult because it involves forming a hypothesis about the underlying or hidden feelings/topics the patient just hints at with his/her statements. Egan says that primary accurate empathy means "sharing hunches about clients and their overt and covert experiences, behaviors and feelings which the therapist thinks will help patients see their problems and concerns more clearly, and in a context that will enable them to move to goal setting and action" (Egan 1982, 79).

Advanced accurate empathy helps the patient in several specific ways. First, it can help him/her become aware of hidden or forbidden feelings. Male patients, for example, often try to hide their sad or hurt feelings because they consider them to be a sign of weakness. Secondly, the therapist can use AAE to help the patient see patterns of behavior or general trends. A bad experience with one doctor, for example, may lead a patient to mistrust all doctors. A third way that AAE can help a patient is to help him or her draw logical conclusions to his or her behaviors or comments. An older teen who feels trapped by his parents' rules and says he's tired of his parents treating him like a child may be expressing a desire to leave home and become more independent. Actually moving out may be very scary to an adolescent who has never been on his own, but that is where his comments seem to be leading.

Since advanced accurate empathy is really the therapist's hypothesis or educated guess about the patient's implications, it is best to present these ideas tentatively. Always leave yourself a way out, by using phrases like "could it be that...," "it seems likely that...," or "I could be wrong, but...." The fact is, you could be wrong, and it should always be acceptable for the patient to correct you if you are. Even if you're not wrong, if the patient really is hiding a seething rage at his spouse, he may not be ready to face or accept such intense feeling. Tentativeness also leaves the patient a way out, without damaging the therapeutic relationship.

The easiest way to learn advanced accurate empathy is to begin with primary accurate empathy. Practice AAE by doing the following exercise.

Advanced Accurate Empathy Worksheet

Directions: First, respond with a primary accurate empathy statement to the patient. Then, respond with some statement of advanced accurate empathy. Freely interpret so as to assist the client in taking a larger view of his or her situation, see the implications or examine the logical conclusions of what is said or done.

1. Sam, age 54
   Situation: This man has a variety of problems. This time he's just undergone surgery to repair a back injury. His tendency is to ruminate constantly on his defects.
   "To feel bad, all I have to do is review what has happened in my life. This past year I let my drinking get the best of me for four months. Over the years, I've messed up my marriage. Now my wife and I are separated. I don't have the kind of income that can support two households, and the job market is really tight. I'm not so sure what skills I have to market anyhow."

Therapist PAE response:

Therapist AAE response:

2. Adele, age 44
   Situation: This woman has been admitted for the third time with a bleeding ulcer.
   "I'm completely depressed. I don't feel like working anymore. Actually I work all the time. I can't think of any day I get up and don't intend to work. I think I begrudge myself the time I take for relaxation. There's been no day for the past two years when I said, 'Today's a day off.' I always feel so good about myself after I've worked hard, and after all, it's my choice to spend the time the way I want, isn't it?"

Therapist PAE response:

Therapist AAE response:

Confrontation

Confrontation involves the resolution of possible discrepancies, distortions, games and smoke screens patients use to avoid self-understanding and/or behavior change. It includes challenging the undeveloped, unused or misused potentialities, skills and resources patients may have as well. Confrontation as a technique is actually an extension of advanced accurate empathy or interpretation. However, whereas interpretation involves the therapist's understanding of a patient's behavior, confrontation permits the patient himself to put his own meaning to the behavior. In confrontation, the therapist points out maladaptive behaviors or inconsistent actions and comments, and invites the patient to explain or make sense of them.

Confrontation has a reputation for being harsh and accusing. However, the skilled confrontation is not harsh, but an act of caring. It should offer genuine feedback to the patient about his comments or behavior, while leaving the judgment of the behavior up to him. The tone of voice used by the therapist is very important here. The correct words, conveyed in an angry or accusing tone, will not achieve the desired result. What is hoped for is self-discovery on the part of the patient, using the confrontation as a guide.

For example, when Ben expresses that he's "happy-go-lucky and able to cope with almost anything," the therapist might ask, "If this is true, what are you doing on an inpatient ward of a psychiatric hospital?" In this confrontation, it is Ben who has to explain the discrepancy between his healthy self-presentation and his psychiatric inpatient status. The therapist might say, "One doesn't get admitted to a psychiatric ward by being healthy and able to cope. How did a healthy person like you end up on a psychiatric ward?" There must be problems Ben isn't talking about. However, the point of the confrontation is not to accuse Ben of having problems; the point is to get Ben himself to stop denying or hiding his problems, and instead try to solve them.

Use the following exercise to practice your skills in confrontation as an act of caring and promoting self-understanding.

Practice in Confrontation Worksheet

Directions: Respond to each of the following clients first with primary accurate empathy, then with confrontation.

Example: Sheila says "Everything is fine." as she stares at the floor and looks sad. Therapist confrontation: You must feel sad, judging from the downcast look on your face. Yet you're telling me everything is fine. How do you see that?

1. Mike, a spinal cord injured patient, age 25, comments after a visit from his wife: "It really hurts me when I think about what she said to me." (He smiles and shrugs his shoulders.)

Therapist confrontation:

2. Anne, age 35, is an arthritic patient who has become socially isolated except for a few friends. She is seeking ways of getting along better with others interpersonally. "I give a lot to my friends, but I expect a lot in return. Unfortunately, it seems like many of them don't recognize my caring and I react by getting angry with them."

Therapist confrontation:

3. Robert, a cardiac patient, is recently divorced, has lost his job and is broke. He keeps joking about it.

Therapist confrontation:

Goals

The goals of groups using the existential/humanistic frame of reference, as mentioned earlier, are self-awareness, self-understanding and self-actualization. These give the OT very clear guidelines about what types of issues need attention. Many aspects of the self can be explored, i.e., feelings and their expression, self-identity and characteristics of the self, style of interaction with others and with groups, body image and feelings about the body, values and attitudes of individuals, and an exploration of the barriers which prevent people from achieving their potential.

Whatever the goal, it is important that it be relevant to the here and now, and applicable to the person's present life situation. Historical causes of difficulty are only a focus in humanistic therapy if they affect present behavior.

Structure

Since the humanistic approach is person-centered, it is best to give minimal structure in occupational therapy groups using this frame of reference. This allows the individual members to have more say about the direction of therapy. Order can be maintained and direction kept clear by providing appropriate activities and limiting the range of choices in the group sessions. As the group is introduced, it is important for the therapist to set ground rules and communicate norms which reflect the basic assumptions of humanistic theory. Respect for one another, non-judgmental acceptance and genuineness are important basic values for the OT to explain and to model.

Examples of Activities

Occupational therapy modalities that are appropriate for this frame of reference are those which promote the goals of existential/humanistic therapy. Issues to be worked on in group activities are: autonomy, love and intimacy, making choices, loneliness and solitude, death and loss, the search for meaning and values, vocational choice and readiness skills, and developing a philosophy to live by (Corey 1986, 96). Creative activities are well suited to these purposes, as well as the practice of specific skills. Some examples of appropriate activities for existential/humanistic groups are listed in the following worksheets.

Self-Awareness Worksheet

Directions: Fill out all the information listed on the worksheet. Then, select what parts you would like to share with the group.

I am (name you prefer):

Some of my needs are:

Some of my hopes are:

I would describe myself as:

Some things that are important in my life *now* are:

Some things that may *become* important to me are:

Three things I'm trying to achieve are:

I am good at:

Some things I'd like to improve about myself are:

I run away from:

I feel confident when:

I am proud of:

My most striking quality is:

Positive Attitudes Worksheet

Materials: Magazines (at least two per patient) with pictures on a variety of subjects.

Directions: Select from these magazines pictures of negative scenes or situations. There is no required number, so find as many as you like. You have fifteen minutes for this task.

Procedure: Each member presents his or her pictures and describes the negative situation. Then the group is asked to point out all the positive aspects of the pictures. For example, appearance or personal hygiene of the people, weather conditions, communication and support available, etc. Then the group can choose a few situations to problem-solve. Answer the question: "What can be done to give this situation a happy ending?"

Leisure Collage Worksheet

Materials: magazines on varied topics, scissors, glue, white paper, markers

Directions: Cut pictures of things you like to do from these magazines and arrange and paste them on the paper. You have 20 minutes to do this task. After you have finished pasting, use a marker to label each picture with a word ending in ''ing.'' Examples are: eating, talking, playing volleyball, singing, etc.

Saying Goodbye Worksheet

Materials: writing paper and pens

Directions: At some point in our lives, we have all had to leave someone we love. Either we left, or we got left behind, i.e., a best friend moving away, a lover finding a new love, a relative's death, a child going away to school. Often we don't have the chance to say the things we want to say before the separation. So here's another chance. Take the next 15 minutes to write a letter to a loved one, telling them the things you'd like them to know. Begin with Dear _____ , and end with some form of goodbye.

My House Worksheet

Materials: worksheets, rulers, colored markers, pencils with erasers and rulers

Directions: Imagine you are going on a one month vacation, and will live in a small house on the beach by yourself. The beach has a path that leads to town where you can buy food or other supplies. Visualize what the house would look like. You arrive in a taxi with your bags. You step onto the deck, unlock the front door and walk in. What would you like to see? Now fill in the floor plan on the worksheet with whatever you would like in your house. Some suggestions are: sofa, bed, dresser, rug, television set, bookshelf with books, refrigerator, stove, washer, dryer, bicycle, sailboat, etc. (Figure 3-1.)

While doing this activity, think about what necessities you'll need and also what items you'd like to help you enjoy your vacation. You may assume there are other people to socialize with at the beach, but they will not be staying with you. You are the only one living in your house.

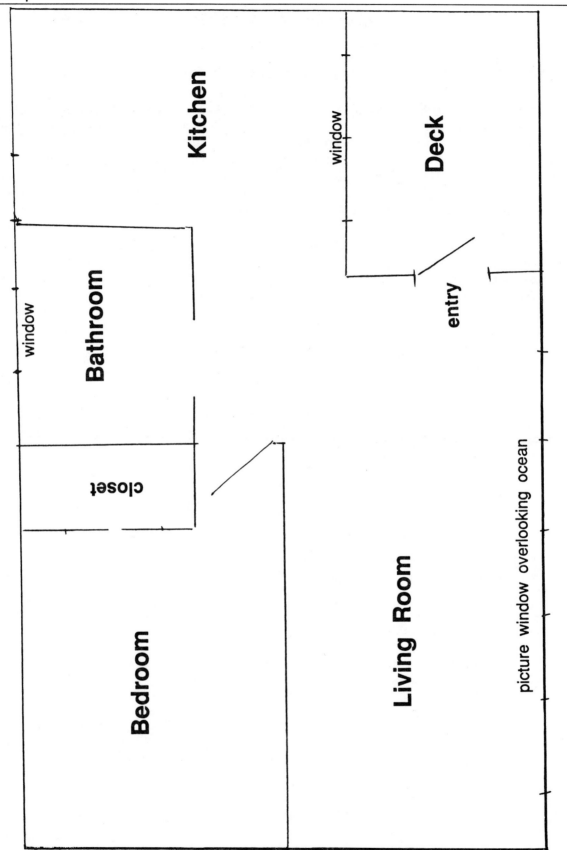

Figure 3-1. "My House" design.

My Ideal Job Worksheet

Materials: worksheets, pencils

Directions: Suppose you had the opportunity to be trained to do whatever job you want. What would be your ideal job? To help you define your ideal job, first write your answers to the following questions. If you circle more than one, write "first" or "second choice" next to the answer.

1. What work setting do you prefer?
   a. contemporary office
   b. well-equipped workshop
   c. home-like setting
   d. outdoors

2. What other people would you prefer to work with?
   a. work by yourself
   b. be part of a working team
   c. be the expert who gives help and advice to others
   d. be your boss's right hand man/woman

3. What skills do you prefer to use while working?
   a. manual skills - work with hands or tools
   b. artistic or creative skills
   c. intellectual skills - knowledge and ideas
   d. political skills - strategies or persuasion
   e. technical problem-solving skills

4. What rewards would you seek from your job?
   a. lots of money
   b. satisfaction from helping others
   c. having others recognize your skills
   d. achieving your own potential

5. How much risk are you willing to take in your job?
   a. prefer doing something familiar with regular pay
   b. don't mind being paid on commission
   c. willing to try new ideas, even if they're not a sure thing
   d. an element of danger might make work more exciting

My Ideal Job Worksheet (continued)

Now consider your answers to those questions and check off the jobs that might fit your critera from the list below:

salesperson in a small clothing store

licensed electrician

mechanic

nursery school teacher

medical technician

nurse in a large hospital

medical receptionist in a doctor's office

advertising artist

newspaper reporter

high school coach

hairdresser

interior decorator

telephone lineman

insurance claims adjuster

traveling salesperson for large company

chef in an expensive restaurant

hostess in an expensive restaurant

manager of a small delicatessen

manager of an expensive antique shop

home health nurse

musician in a band

public relations representative for a hotel

counselor in a drug rehabilitation center

landscape designer

Group Leadership

The general group format presented in Chapter 1 is based on an existential/humanistic approach. Therefore, the seven steps remain basically the same.

Introduction

The sequence is as described in Chapter 1. The therapist gives his or her name and the title of the group followed by acknowledgement/introduction of each member. The environment should facilitate group confidentiality, trust and safety, i.e., a private, soundproof room with a door that closes, free of interruptions for the time allotted.

The warm-up should be carefully selected to reflect therapeutic norms, such as respect and caring for one another, a focus on feelings and open self-disclosure.

Expectations for a group in the existential/humanistic frame of reference will be high, since it assumes that members have the capacity to understand and resolve their own problems without directive intervention from the therapist. This approach is generally not appropriate for patients who are cognitively impaired.

In humanistic groups, the purpose should be thoroughly explained, since member self-understanding and insight is assumed to be possible. Care in this initial explanation will make it possible for the members themselves to strive to accomplish the purpose as they do the activity.

The time frame for the group should allow for longer, more complex and thought-provoking activities. A greater proportion of time in these groups should be set aside for discussion and group interaction. Perhaps 90 minutes or even two hours would not be too long for groups in a humanistic frame of reference.

Activity

Selecting activities is guided by the therapeutic goals of the existential/humanistic frames. The goals are self-awareness, self-understanding and self-actualization. Thus, exploring interests, making choices and developing new skills are also fair game, as long as these activities are patient-directed. Creative activities like drawing, painting, sculpting and storytelling or drama often encourage the expression of hidden aspects of the self, and are helpful in the goals of self-awareness and insight. The therapist selects and structures the activity to maximize goal achievement.

For example, she might choose to have the group draw a "circle of feelings." This requires each member to draw a circle in the center of a piece of 9"x12" white drawing paper. Then they use colored markers to indicate layers of feelings. The outer edge of the circle represents the outer self, the feelings they show to others, while the center of the circle represents the inner core, those feelings kept well-hidden and seldom shown to others. Such an activity serves to focus and guide the group toward a frank discussion of their inner feelings, promoting the goal of greater self-understanding among members.

The time frame for such an activity should adhere to the rule of no more than one third of the entire group time. Emphasis in this frame of reference should always be on discussion and processing.

Sharing

Considerable time should be taken with this stage to be sure each member's work is correctly understood and explored by the group. The therapist might ask questions of each member to help clarify and focus their issues. Leader skills in concreteness, primary accurate empathy, immediacy, confrontation, and advanced accurate empathy can be used effectively in all of the discussion stages of humanistic groups. The occupational therapist can use patient issues as examples to demonstrate the techniques of reality testing and consensual validation for the group. In the humanistic frame of reference, feedback is the most vital therapeutic tool available, and should be encouraged early in groups, beginning in the sharing stage. The purpose of feedback goes beyond the acknowledgement of member contributions. It is a skill to be taught to all the group members if they are to help one another.

In our example of the circle of feelings exercise, members may question one another about the meaning of color and about reported feelings. They may agree or disagree about the outer circle a patient describes. If Ben draws an outer circle of yellow, and reports feeling that others see him as cheerful and carefree, the statement invites other group members to comment. Some may agree with Ben, that he presents a jovial exterior. Others may see beyond this, to his inner pain and suffering. Ben and the group both benefit from a discussion of how he really comes across to others.

Processing

The potential of members sharing the leadership of groups is maximized in the humanistic frame of reference. Thus, the skill of giving and receiving feedback is further defined in the processing stage. As members discuss their feelings about the activity, the leader encourages them to also express feelings about one another. The best that we hope for is a genuine curiosity about one another, leading to concern and caring in the later stages of group development. The focus on feelings in the processing stage is consistent with the humanistic frame of reference. The therapist can further apply this frame by getting members to use their own experiences and capabilities to help one another.

Generalizing

In existential/humanistic theory, the meaning of life is a central concern. The generalizing stage of the group is devoted to deriving the meaning of a small slice of life, the group experience. The therapist should encourage the members to verbalize the meaning of the experience for them. Looking at similarities and differences in what is meaningful will help reinforce the values of each member. Using our "circle of feelings" example again, some members might find meaning in becoming more aware of their own inner feelings, while others might value the opportunity to learn how others really see them. It may surprise some members to find themselves able to express feelings verbally, while others may be more guarded and unwilling to trust their inner feelings to others. Some people seek the understanding of others through self-disclosure and these people find meaning in close relationships with others. For other people, the impression they leave with others might be more important, the "never let them see you sweat" approach. Therapists need to be careful not to judge any value as right or wrong. Accepting differences among members is an important norm to promote in this stage.

Application

In this phase, meaning is expanded and personalized. In humanistic groups, action is not the emphasis. So, the group experience will more likely be applied to the enhancement of self-concept or deeper insight rather than the changing of behavior.

Summary

The summary, as with every phase, should involve the group members whenever possible. They are presumed capable of analyzing the entire group experience and judging which parts are most significant. The therapist's role is to encourage them to do this, and not to do it for them. When the therapist asks for a summary of the group, about five minutes before it's time to end, members will quickly learn that this is what is expected, and may eventually do it spontaneously.

Bibliography

Corey G. *The Theory and Practice of Counseling and Psychotherapy*. 4th ed. Monterey, CA: Brooks/Cole, 1991.

Corey G. *I Never Knew I Had a Choice*. 3rd ed. Monterey, CA: Brooks/Cole, 1986.

Egan G. *Exercises in Helping Skills*. Monterey, CA: Brooks/Cole, 1982.

Egan G. *The Skilled Helper*. 3rd ed. Monterey, CA: Brooks/Cole, 1986.

Huber C. Counseling Techniques. Presentation at University of Bridgeport Department of Graduate Psychology, 1981.

Maddi S.R. *Personality Theories: A Comparative Analysis*. 4th ed. Homewood, IL: The Dorsey Press, 1980.

Maslow A.H. *Toward a Psychology of Being*. Rev. ed. NY: Van Nostrand Reinhold, 1968.

May R. *The Meaning of Anxiety*. Rev. ed. NY: Norton, 1977

May R. and Yalom I. Existential Psychotherapy. (in Corsini R.J. & Wedding D. *Current Psychotherapies*, 4th ed. 1989. pp 363-402, Itasca, IL: F.E. Peacock).

Mosey A.C. *Occupational Therapy: Configuration of a Profession*. NY: Raven Press, 1981.

Mosey A.C. The proper focus of scientific inquiry in occupational therapy: Frames of reference. *Occupational Therapy J of Res*, 1989, 9,4,195-201.

Simon S. *Values Clarification*. NY: Hart Pub., 1972

Smith H. and Hopkins, H., eds. *Willard and Spackman's Occupational Therapy*. 6th ed. Philadelphia: Lippincott, 1983.

Yalom I. *The Theory and Practice of Group Psychotherapy*. 3rd ed. NY: Basic Books, Inc., 1985.

Chapter

4

A Psychoanalytic Approach

For some time now, occupational therapy theorists have been acknowledging the usefulness of various forms of psychoanalytic theory in guiding our treatment of patients with mental illness. Diasio (1968) explores the psychoanalytic view of motivation and the environment. The Fidlers (1963) point out the importance of the unconscious and view activities as part of a communication process with human and non-human objects to effectively gratify instinctual needs. Mosey (1986), in considering analytical frames of reference, emphasizes the "structure for linking psychoanalytic theories, the symbolic potential and reality aspects of activities, and the process of altering intrapsychic content in the direction of providing a more adaptive basis for interaction with the environment." Llorens (1966), refers to "socially acceptable, ego-adaptive functioning" in describing the effect of patient involvement in activity groups, thus focusing on occupational therapy techniques that help develop and strengthen the functions of the ego. Following these early theorists, two general goals of occupational therapy groups will be considered: alteration of personality and development of ego skills. This chapter will first review the basic assumptions of psychoanalytic theory which are useful in planning occupational therapy groups. Ego functions and their relevance to occupational therapy will then be reviewed. Finally, contributions from the occupational therapy literature will be summarized, and group leadership guidelines will be derived from these psychoanalytic theoretical concepts.

Psychoanalytic Theory

Psychoanalytic theory, based on the work of Sigmund Freud in the late 19th and early 20th centuries, has had a profound influence on all theories of group treatment. Corey (1991) describes Freud as an "intellectual giant" whose work represents "the most comprehensive theory of personality and psychotherapy ever developed." In the 1990s, there is a tendency to underestimate the influence of psychoanalytic theory because many subsequent theorists have either developed it further or reacted against it. The current emphasis on brain biochemistry as a determinant of human behavior has overshadowed the importance of personality dynamics in our understanding of mental illness. New technology has enabled researchers to observe the physiological and biochemical functioning of the brain in ways never before possible, and thus new genetic links have been discovered.

However, for occupational therapists, these new scientific discoveries do not alter the fact that there are many mental illnesses currently being diagnosed for which psychoanalytic theory offers the only plausible explanation. For example, there is a growing interest in borderline personality disorder, which is thought to originate from a failure to separate from parents and achieve an autonomous sense of self at around age two. If the parent does not allow the child to explore his environment and do activities of his own choosing in a safe environment, then as an adult, he is unable to derive any satisfaction from activities. Knowing this, the occupational therapist can offer patients with borderline personality disorder an opportunity to explore activities according to their own interest. Recent research shows that for some borderline patients, it is possible to strengthen autonomous functioning through participation in task-oriented occupational therapy groups (Greene & Cole 1991).

For occupational therapists, psychoanalytic theory is also useful in the physical disability areas of practice. The concept of self-worth and the many defenses of the ego can help us understand why some of our patients use denial of their illness, or resist our suggestions for treatment. It is important for occupational therapists to determine the symbolic meaning of illness or trauma in the structure of personality, and how symptoms are incorporated into the patient's perception of herself. For example, Julia, an 83-year-old woman with osteoporosis and chronic arthritis, was in and out of doctors' offices all her life, with many failed attempts to increase her independent functioning in occupational therapy. Only at age 79, after her husband died, did she learn to perform self-care independently. In her earlier years, Julia's many illnesses symbolized her helplessness. Her dependency on her husband for personal self-care fulfilled her need for attention and love. The patient's sense of self is vital to her acceptance or rejection of occupational therapy treatment, whether the illness is mental or physical.

The original form of psychoanalytic theory, sometimes called "id psychology" (Fine 1979, 319) has been widely criticized by psychologists, social scientists and occupational therapists during the last twenty years for its vagueness and its unsuitability for research. The link with psychoanalysis and its questionable appropriateness for treating many types of mental illness has added fuel to the fires of discontent. Psychoanalysis is a therapeutic approach developed by Freud, in which individual patients are assisted in uncovering their unconscious conflicts by conversing with a therapist, a process which could take many years. Critics feel that one cannot research the unconscious, since it is not observable or measurable.

A more current emphasis on ego psychology focuses on the conscious rather than the unconscious aspects of the personality and is therefore, by definition, more observable and measurable. The **ego** is best understood as the "self." A patient's sense of self, his self-concept, can determine his degree of involvement in occupational therapy treatment. If a patient sees himself as a capable and worthwhile individual, he will be motivated to overcome disability. If Dean defines himself as an accountant, he will make the effort to overcome his depression to return to that occupation. In this frame of reference, the ego is seen as a powerful motivating force which can either resist or facilitate therapeutic change.

Bellak (1973) operationalized the functions of the ego, making them more amenable for research purposes. He defines twelve ego functions: 1) reality testing, 2) judgment, 3) sense of self and the world, 4) control of drive, affect and impulse, 5) object relationships, 6) thought processes, 7) adaptive regression in service of the ego, 8) defensive functioning, 9) stimulus barrier, 10) autonomous functioning, 11) synthetic integrative functions and 12) mastery/competence. These functions most applicable to occupational therapy will be further defined later in this chapter.

Basic Assumptions

The following is intended as a brief review of the original concepts of Freudian psychoanalytic theory. A more thorough understanding may be obtained by referring to other basic psychology texts. Psychoanalytic theory is exceedingly complex, and there are many variations currently in use. It must be remembered that Freud's theory provides an *intellectual* understanding of the personality and its development. The parts described as id, ego and superego do not parallel structures or functions of the brain, nor do they represent distinct developmental stages. The purpose for which psychoanalytic theory will be used in this text is to define those concepts which help us understand the dynamics of illness, both mental and physical, and to develop treatment techniques to address these dynamics. Because of the focus on group treatment, many important aspects of Freudian theory will be left out.

Personality Structure

Freud organized personality into three parts: the id, the ego and the superego. This structure is still accepted by many psychotherapists regardless of their discipline or theoretical preferences. While a balance of these components is considered ideal, the functions of the ego in this text will be emphasized because of their direct relevance to occupational therapy groups.

The Id

The id is seen as largely unconscious. It is the part of the personality which houses primitive drives and instincts, needs and conflicts, that the ego is unable to integrate. The id is the biological component of the personality, and is thought to operate through primary process thinking. Primary process thinking is the earliest to develop in the infant. It is illogical and undisciplined and operates on the pleasure principle, demanding immediate gratification of needs and drives.

The Ego

The ego is the psychological component and has contact with the external world. It functions logically and works to achieve a balance between internal drives and external expectations. The ego operates through a secondary process, one that is learned through experience in reaching compromises and applying logic and discipline in an attempt to adapt to the environment.

The Superego

The superego is the social component of the personality which serves as an individual's moral code, his sense of good and bad, right and wrong. The superego is often illogical and unrealistic in its quest for idealism and perfection. The superego is the last part to appear in the developmental process and its beliefs are learned from parents and from society.

Psychosexual Stages

Freud believed that personality is largely determined by one's early childhood experiences. Psychosexual stages of development, spanning a range of 18 years from birth to maturity, are differentiated by changes in the objects which potentially provide need satisfaction. An object is someone or something that which gratifies or frustrates a need; objects can be human or non-human. The classic example of an object in the oral stage is mother's breast. A non-human substitute for mother's breast is the bottle. When a child's needs are gratified, he thrives and is able to develop and move on to the next stage. However, when the child's needs are continually frustrated, he develops a fixation which can remain in the unconscious and cause many of the problems in adulthood which we know as symptoms of illness. Freud's psychosexual stages of development are outlined in Table 4-1.

The psychosexual stages are critical to our understanding of mental illness. In spite of current discoveries of the genetic and biochemical origins of some illnesses, most psychopathology is still explained in terms of Freud's levels of personality organization. In general, the earlier the conflict occurs, the more severe the illness. While there are not rigid parallels between the stages and the development of certain illnesses, fixations in the early stages are likely to result in faulty or incomplete development in later ones. For example, failure to develop self-control in the anal stage may result in the over-development or misuse of defense mechanisms as the ego's attempt to compensate for lack of self-control in later stages.

When we, as occupational therapists, observe patients in our therapeutic groups who are unable to work together and get along with one another, a knowledge of how the patients have progressed through the psychosexual stages may help us understand the reasons why. In addition, the stages may offer guidelines as to what type of therapeutic intervention is needed. For example, trust is an issue dealt with in the oral stage. Groups in which members seem to lack a basic trust of one another might benefit from activities which assist patients in feeling more comfortable with self-disclosure. This self-disclosure can form the basis of establishing trusting relationships with the therapist and with one another.

Psychic Energy, Libido, Aggression and Anxiety

In Freud's view, the amount of psychic energy is limited, and must be shared by all three parts of the personality. This explains why people cease to function when too much

Table 4-1. Freud's Psychosexual Stages		
Age (years)	**Stage (source of gratification)**	**Fixation Characteristics (potential problem areas)**
Birth-1 year	*Oral Stage* early - sucking late - biting	Theme: trust, dependency Regression: psychosis
1-3 years	*Anal Stage* early - excreting late - retaining	Theme: control, autonomy Regression: neurosis, character disorders
3-5 years	*Phallic Stage* genital interest penis envy	Theme: Oedipal/Electra complex
5-12 years	*Latency Stage* sublimation of sexual drive superego develops	Theme: Skill development social role development emergence of guilt
11-adulthood	*Genital Stage* puberty capacity for intimacy	Theme: Sexual identity adult responsibility for love and work

energy is being used up in trying to deal with unresolved conflicts from the past. A healthy individual is able to resolve conflicts as they arise and therefore keep psychic energy available for the ego to grow and develop, and interact effectively with the environment. In mental illness, psychic energy may be trapped in the id and may produce non-adaptive behaviors which we call symptoms.

Two specific forms of psychic energy are described by Freud, the libidinal and the aggressive drives. Libido is the sexual energy which represents the urge to perpetuate life, to be intimate, to love and to reproduce. This is also called the life-force, and is demonstrated by a person's tendency to form relationships with other people. The aggressive drive is equated with the death-force, and is associated with hostility, hatred and the urge to destroy. It is expressed in the tendency to be self-sufficient and to keep others at a distance. Both the libidinal and the aggressive drives are part of the id, and both seek expression through objects. It is a function of the ego to control these drives and to allow their expression in ways that are socially acceptable. It is a function of the superego to guide an individual's libidinal and aggressive drives toward constructive and morally acceptable expression.

Anxiety, in Freud's view, is defined in relation to both drives and the ego's control function. Anxiety is an alerting response which lets us know that something is wrong and needs to be changed and that some action needs to be taken to get us out of danger. However, unlike the existentialists who view anxiety as a normal condition of life, Freud views anxiety as pathological. Freudian anxiety develops out of the conflicts over control of the available psychic energy within the personality itself. This anxiety goes beyond fear of realistic danger from the external world. It is the fear that the id may take over, forcing the individual to act irrationally or in ways that are morally wrong, or that the superego may take over, causing a pervasive sense of guilt and self-punishment. As long as the ego maintains control, anxiety can be safely held in check and dealt with realistically. High levels of neurotic anxiety, however, may necessitate the unconscious use of ego defense mechanisms to help reduce the tension and protect the survival of the ego. These mechanisms will be reviewed later in this chapter.

Occupational therapists may facilitate the expression of psychic energy through activities. This helps the patient in a variety of ways. Through activities, the aggressive drive can be directed toward productive work, constructive homemaking or toward competition in sports. The libidinal drive can energize the patient to development of social skills, nurturing skills and cooperation with others. Various ego functions might be encouraged in occupational therapy groups, such as appropriate expression of feelings, both loving and aggressive, or the sharing of perceptions to help members develop a realistic sense of self.

Symbols, Projections and Communication with the Unconscious

Rarely, except in episodes of psychosis, does the content of the unconscious become known. Psychoanalytic therapy's main thrust is to help an individual become aware of his unconscious conflicts and fixations, so that the mature ego can deal with them effectively and resolve them. However, the nature of primary process makes awareness of unconscious material very complex. Primary process is not organized or logical, and is not remembered in words or complete thoughts. Highly emotional material may take the form of symbols which represent experiences which originally produced them. For example, a child who experienced the violent death of a parent in an automobile accident, may have repressed the original memory. If as an adult, he draws a car as part of an occupational therapy activity, he may suddenly reexperience an overwhelming feeling of grief and loss without knowing why. It is the therapist's role to help the adult patient to interpret the meaning of the symbols he produces, and with the help of a psychiatrist, remember and work through the original traumatic experience.

Object Relationships

Object relationships were previously mentioned as the organizing principles of the psychosexual stages. Freud viewed object relations as the foundation of an individual's capacity to love and to work. The Fidlers (1963) define occupational therapy in terms of the development of relationships with human (therapist) and non-human (environment) objects. In human relationships, the patient develops the ability to satisfy some of his basic needs, such as recognition, self-esteem and belonging, through a therapeutic relationship with the occupational therapist. In the safety of a therapeutic environment, the patient uses realistic feedback from the therapist or other patients to correct his unrealistic concepts and expectations of self and others. Non-human objects are related to the patient's ability to work. The patient can learn, in occupational therapy, to use the symbolic as well as actual properties of objects to help satisfy instinctual drives and needs. For example, Bob can satisfy his need to express hostility by flattening a ball of clay, or sawing a piece of wood. Mary can express her compulsive needs by maintaining a perfectly clean and organized kitchen. Using this principle, occupational therapy activities can be selected according to the instinctual needs of group members.

Assumptions of Ego Psychology

Alfred Adler (Fine 1979) is credited with making the first significant break with Freud over the nature and importance of the ego. He believed that the ego is responsible for shaping the personality, rather than the person being shaped by biological forces and early childhood experiences. Another theorist who recognized the importance of the ego was Heinz Hartmann. Hartmann (1939) looked at the process of psychoanalysis and suggested that it was not a reconstruction of what once existed buried in the unconscious (the Freudian view). He saw that psychotherapy requires that the mature ego establish correct causal relationships and judgments of the emerging memories. The significance of Hartmann's work is in establishing the autonomy of the ego as separate from the id in psychoanalytic theory. Ego psychology has been developing since 1923, and has had many spokesmen, including Adler, Sullivan, Hartmann, Erikson, Lewin and Rapaport (Fine 1979). The common element is an emphasis on the ego. For the sake of brevity, not all the functions of the ego can be reviewed. Those selected for emphasis are reality testing, sense of self, thought processes, judgment, self-control, defensive mechanisms and competence/mastery.

Reality Testing

Reality testing is perhaps the most important function of the ego in therapy. It is the ego's ability to use perception and judgment to differentiate between internal needs and external demands. This process involves the use of interaction with the environment and with others in shaping and reshaping one's views of self and the world. It is precisely this process which is responsible for adaptation to the environment. The ego becomes aware of needs and drives from the id, but delays their gratification until they can be satisfied in ways that are socially acceptable.

Consensual Validation

Reality testing is an integral part of the therapeutic use of groups. As members share their perceptions of themselves and the world with others in the group, they have the advantage of hearing the responses of others. It is through this feedback that group members gather evidence to support their self-other perceptions. When perceptions of others are clearly different from one's own, then one needs to question whether her own perceptions are realistic. The process of integrating one's own perceptions, views or beliefs with those of others is called consensual validation.

For example, Lisa shared with the group a painful experience involving her father's rejection of her. Lisa believed she had to live with this rejection and was powerless to change it. Several other members recounted similar feelings about their own fathers, based on similar experiences. This feedback helped validate Lisa's feelings of rejection; based on clear evidence, she had a right to feel rejected—in her situation, anyone would. However, another member of the group, Roberta, also told Lisa how she had begun speaking to her father after a seven year period of silence. Roberta was able to significantly improve her father-daughter relationship through some more adult conversations and sharing of feelings. This feedback made Lisa reconsider her position; perhaps she was not as powerless as she believed herself to be. The group helped Lisa to see which parts of her self-perception were real (being rejected) and which were not real (being powerless).

Exploring Outer Reality

Occupational therapy groups involving the use of concrete tasks provide another kind of reality testing, one on a sensory level. Manipulation of objects and materials provides sensory input: taste, touch, smell, vision, hearing and proprioception (position, pressure, balance, etc.), which can lead on to challenge internal perceptions. Robert felt he had no energy and therefore could not complete a woodworking project. When the group members persuaded him to try it, however, the sensory stimulation provided by sawing and hammering the wood (proprioceptive and auditory), helped release the needed energy. Robert learned through experience that by engaging in appropriate motor activities, he was able to direct his energy to produce a positive effect on the environment (a completed project). If the group then also provides positive feedback on his wood project, Robert is further inclined to change his view of himself from ineffectual, "I can't" to effective, "I can!" It is important here for the occupational therapist to be aware of Robert's abilities in choosing a task, ensuring that his experience is likely to be a successful one.

Sense of Self

Many aspects of sense of self appear in the literature, and their meaning can be somewhat confusing. Three discrete aspects will be defined here: self-concept, body image and self-esteem.

Self-Concept

Self-concept or self-identity is sometimes used interchangeably with the word *ego*. Developmentally, the idea of self originates when the infant begins to differentiate self from mother, and then from the environment in general. Psychotic individuals are understood by ego psychologists to have regressed beyond the point where they are able to differentiate self from others. These psychotic individuals are said to have "poor" or "loose" ego boundaries. This factor makes psychotic patients particularly sensitive to their environment. When someone in the group is angry, for example, it is often the psychotic patient who is first to notice it, although he may not express his awareness realistically or appropriately.

Following Freud's original formulations, the attempt was made to correlate the various clinical entities with the points of fixation in psychosexual development. Primarily, the oral stage is associated with psychosis, the anal stage with neuroses, and the phallic stage with hysteria. Ego psychologists have elaborated and changed this original oversimplified concept of mental illness, but have retained the idea that the ego or self-concept is fundamentally different in these three levels of psychiatric diagnosis. Psychological testing such as word association (Jung 1906), interpretation of inkblots (Rorschach 1921) and association with photographs (Murray's Thematic Apperception Test 1935) are a few of the earliest attempts to measure ego functions with particular regard to self-concept.

The idea that concept of the self is a common problem area for mentally ill individuals has lead occupational therapists to make self-concept and its related ideas, body image, self-esteem and self-perception, the focus of occupational therapy treatment. Groups using movement or dance, or physical sports and exercise may be helpful to patients in developing a realistic body image. Drawing and word association activities, often taking their cue from the various psychological tests, have been useful in promoting knowledge of the self. Self-esteem is better approached in occupational therapy through successful experiences and feedback from others. Person drawings in particular, are a useful therapeutic tool, for both evaluation and treatment in occupational therapy.

Body Image

Body image is the perception of one's physical self that forms the basis of self-awareness. According to theories of child development, the earliest learning involves the association and differentiation of somatosensory sensations. These provide a kind of geographical knowledge of the body and how it works that defines "me." Body sense, according to Allport (1958), allows a child to develop a sense of personhood. It is the sensory motor exploration of early play that helps the child define the boundaries of his body and distinguish "me" from "not me." In adulthood, body sense continues to provide a basic reference point from which environmental interactions take place. The sensory systems, for example, help people know how they feel. Influences from the body guide day to day behavior. For example, you may stay home from work because you feel fatigued, or you may go for a walk because you feel restless. The child achieves a sense of control over his body by reaching out to the environment to satisfy body needs: a bottle satisfies hunger, a toy satisfies need for pleasure, mother satisfies the need for comfort. As adults, we continue to reach out to the environment and to others, based on our perceptions of our bodies and what we need.

Illness tends to produce distortions in body image, and this may be the source of problem behaviors. As occupational therapists, one of our goals is to determine whether our patient's body image is realistic. Using activities that encourage patients to become aware of their feelings and sensations can help to correct body image distortions. Movement activities and person drawings are two examples of this.

Self-Esteem

Self-esteem describes the subjective feelings of one's own ability. As with sensory motor, perceptual and cognitive processes, feelings are innate and develop as the child matures. However, feelings or affects are intricately tied to objects, and their expression determines how people relate to one another and to their world. The idea that affects are ego states comes from Freud's 1926 work *Inhibitions, Symptoms and Anxiety*. Rapaport (1953) attempted to articulate a theory of affect, suggesting that affect originates as psychic energy and is seen as a signal emitted by the ego to indicate an internal feeling state needing to be noticed. Spitz (1959) offered a theory of affect development in the infant as 1) crying, 2) smiling and 3) stranger distress or fearfulness. Language development then allows the child to express a multiplicity of feeling states of increasing complexity.

The expression of affect or emotion is an important function of the ego. As suggested by Rapaport, it is one of the ways the ego has to control and direct energy from the id. Acting out has been described earlier as a more primitive, less socialized form of expression of affect through action. Those with special talents are able to express affect through artistic media, such as painting, music or poetry and drama. While these ways are socially acceptable, the most commonly acceptable way to express affect is by describing it verbally with words.

As occupational therapists, we often observe in our patients (and sometimes in ourselves) a lack of ability to communicate emotions to others. In the ego adaptive frame of reference, a common goal of occupational therapy groups is the appropriate expression of emotions.

Thought Processes

Thought processes are the cognitive functions of the ego having to do with attention, memory, learning and logical thought, compromise, problem solving and judgment.

Attention

Attention is the ability of the ego to focus on something for a period of time. It requires not only alertness of the mind, but a readiness to take in new information. Information coming in through the sensory systems is screened for relevance and the brain focuses on aspects of the environment to which a response is appropriate. Sustained attention, or concentration, is needed for the individual to participate in occupational therapy groups.

Memory

Memory is central to psychoanalytic theory, as seen in Freud's persistent efforts to recapture early childhood events. Rapaport (1942) recognized the relationship between memory and emotional factors. The ego was thought to censor memory in accordance with the intensity of associated emotional factors. In other words, events that were extremely painful are repressed; the ego stores them below the level of consciousness and they cannot be remembered at all. Or, the ego can alter the perception of a traumatic event, so that the senses are numbed and the brain will not receive more stimuli than it can handle. In this case, the memory of the event would be inaccurate or unrealistic. The current metaphor most closely associated with memory is that of the computer, with information storage and retrieval as the primary activities. It is believed that one's memory process reflects individual styles of secondary process functioning. In other words, what someone remembers is dependent upon how he perceives and understands an event in the first place.

When an occupational therapist hears a patient report a remembered event in a group, it becomes the task of the therapist to listen not only for the facts, but also for the emotional bias the patient expresses. This is particularly important if the patient's emotional response is problematic. For example, Shelley reported at the beginning of the group that something about the last group had been bothering her all week. Last week, during a serious discussion among several group members, Shelley had gotten up from her chair and stepped into the center of the group to kill a spider that was crawling on the floor. She felt "terrible" that her action would be viewed as a violation or mocking of the members whose discussion she had disrupted. The group's response to this confession was surprising. Two or three members remembered the incident in passing, but said it was "no big deal." The three members who were involved in the discussion had no recall of the event at all—just as though it never happened. The facts of the spider killing event were the same for everyone, but Shelley remembered them in the context to a strong emotional bias which put herself in a negative light. It was only with the feedback of the other group members that she was able to shed the bias and put the event in a more realistic perspective.

With most significant events in our lives, we do not have the advantage of the feedback of the others to help us correct our emotional bias. Hence when past events not witnessed by the group are reported to the group, it is difficult for members or the therapist to separate the facts from the emotions involved. It is only in the context of "here and now" events that groups can be helpful in this way. This is one reason that it is suggested that our occupational therapy groups have a "here and now" focus.

Learning and Logical Thought

Learning is a skill of the ego which has been given little attention by followers of psychoanalysis; yet it is central to the notion of making therapeutic change. It has been noted by ego psychologists (1950) that intellectual development (learning) occurs most favorably in a warm, secure environment. This observation is helpful to occupational therapy so we can recognize the importance of creating and maintaining this kind of safe environment in our groups. Physical safety should be a given; this means that the OT removes any dangerous objects or factors from the environment, i.e., sharp objects, loose wires, wet or slippery floors. Psychological safety is provided when the occupational therapist maintains control through the establishment of group norms, such as mutual respect and prevention of verbal attacks on one another.

The kind of thinking attributed to the ego is secondary process thinking. This is also called reasoning or logical thought. It is the ability of the ego to consider facts in the light of reality and put them to use in guiding behavior. Problem-solving is a cognitive skill which requires the use of logical thought. In fact, all of the functions of the ego contribute to problem-solving: accurate perception and reality testing, memory and control of impulses as well as appropriate use of defenses. The process of solving problems is quite complex, but the ability to do so is often a deciding factor in whether our patients are considered to be competent in activities of daily living. Occupational therapists are often asked to evaluate a patient's problem-solving ability. Observation of the patient in a group activity is one way to determine this skill. For example, Rich, a patient in a cooking group, was unfamiliar with the process of peeling and slicing carrots for a salad. However, since he had arrived late, that was the only job available. Rich picked up the knife and proceeded to chop the carrot, leaving the skin on and cutting only part way through with each chop. When another patient handed Rich a vegetable peeler, Rich turned on the would-be helper and waved the knife at him in a somewhat threatening way. After a few more attempts to cut the skin off the carrot with the knife, Rich put down the carrot and abandoned the task. After observing Rich's behavior, the occupational therapist discussed the situation with Rich and determined that Rich's ability to solve problems was poor.

How can occupational therapy groups be helpful to Rich in learning to solve problems? Clearly, teaching him to use a vegetable peeler will only help temporarily in the specific situation. In general, Rich's tendency to act alone and reject help are the real issues that need to be dealt with. Group discussion following the cooking task helped Rich to understand what his options were in solving the carrot problem. Asking for help and being able to accept it in a non-threatening way were agreed upon as goals for Rich in future group tasks.

Judgment

Judgment is another function of the ego which is often the focus in occupational therapy groups. Good judgment requires the following cognitive processes: accurate and realistic perception of the situation, identification of intended behaviors and likely consequences, prediction of the behaviors' effect on others, control of response until options are considered, and an appreciation of what it takes to accomplish something. On a well-known psychological test, the patient is asked the question, "What is the thing to do if you find an envelope in the street that is sealed, addressed and has a new stamp?" The most acceptable answer is "mail it" (Wechsler 1981, 126). How one arrives at this response requires a complex process of perception, reasoning and anticipation of consequences. Judgment is a cognitive skill of the highest order, and one of the most difficult to learn or teach.

Self Control

Control was the earliest of the ego functions to be recognized, when Freud conceptualized the ego's main function to control the instinctual drives from the id. Impulse control may be seen as a derivative of this earlier conceptualization.

In occupational therapy groups, we often encourage impulse control in a number of ways. We expect group members to arrive on time, and to remain attentive for the length of the group, usually 50-60 minutes. We expect members to consider others in the group, listening to them, waiting their turn to speak, sharing tools and materials, passing the glue or the scissors. In a cooking group, we would ask members not to taste the food with their fingers, and to wait to begin eating until the whole group is seated. On a shopping trip, we ask our patients not to taste items in the store, not to buy items impulsively and to wait to light their cigarette until they have finished shopping. Following social norms and interacting effectively in groups requires good control of impulses.

Defense Mechanisms

Defenses are broadly understood as a way of warding off anxiety and ensuring the safety and preservation of an intact ego. The strengthening of healthy defenses is a common goal in occupational therapy groups. In addition, the concept of defenses helps us as occupational therapists to understand better our patient's response to activities. Through our recognition of defenses in our patients, we as occupational therapists are better able to plan activities and make therapeutic interventions in our groups to help patients achieve a healthy balance in their lives.

Defense mechanisms are an important part of the structure of the ego. Early psychologists focused on this aspect when developing the techniques of psychoanalysis. The goal of psychoanalysis was to break through a persons defenses so as to uncover the memory of critical childhood events.

Kaplan and Sadock (1988) have classified defense mechanisms into four categories:
1. Narcissistic defenses: projection, denial and distortion;
2. Immature defenses: acting out, blocking, hypochondriasis, introjection, passive-aggressive behavior, projection, regression, schizoid fantasy, somatization and turning against the self;
3. Neurotic defenses: controlling, displacement, dissociation, externalization, inhibition, intellectualization, isolation, rationalization, reaction formation, repression, sexualization and undoing;
4. Mature defenses: altruism, anticipation, asceticism, humor, sublimation and suppression.

The contemporary ego psychologists view mature defenses as performing a healthy adaptive function, and these will be most relevant to our work in occupational therapy. Those defenses which are dealt with most often in occupational therapy are reviewed here. The reader is referred to Kaplan and Sadock (1988) for a more thorough description of the above defenses.

Sublimination

Sublimation was identified by Anna Freud in 1936 as a healthy and acceptable rechanneling of libidinal and aggressive drives into constructive activity. While sublimation is no longer a focus in psychological literature, the concept remains central to occupational therapy because of its implications regarding activity, creativity and tasks or work. As occupational therapists using a psychoanalytic frame of reference, we continue to see clear evidence of this rechanneling of energy. The concept allows us to understand why work is such a central part of living, and why the loss of the work role produces both aggressiveness and anxiety, and a sharp decline in one's self-worth. Neuturalization (Hartmann's updated substitute for sublimation) refers to the de-energizing of the libidinal and aggressive drives. It is the "successful defense" by which the mature ego masters reality.

Projection

Projection is another defense, originating with Freud (1911) which continues to hold value in occupational therapy. The modern day variation was described by Melanie Klein (1948) as projective identification. In this mechanism, parts of the self are split off and projected onto an external object or person. Projection provides the ego with a means of getting rid of bad parts of the self. Sam is angry with his boss, but he believes the anger is bad, so he projects the anger onto his boss. Now Sam can like himself and feel justified in believing his boss is the bad guy who gets angry. Good parts of the self may be projected also, to avoid separation or keep them safe from the bad parts. Projection at higher levels leads to misinterpreting the motives, feelings, attitudes or intentions of others.

Projection as a concept is used extensively in occupational therapy in the form of projective techniques. Projective techniques are generally creative modalities such as drawing, sculpture, poetry, creative writing or drama, which allow/encourage a person to express the hidden parts of the self. A patient is said to project parts of himself, particularly affects such as anger or love, in the form of symbols or shapes in art or characters and situations in writing or drama. When done in adulthood, these images or fantasies are then open to interpretation by the mature ego. As therapists, we encourage our patients to apply logic and mature judgment to the products of their projective creations when we ask them to explain them to their fellow group members. One Vietnam veteran participating in an occupational therapy projective arts group was asked to explain his elaborate drawing of the atrocities of war. The guns, the dead body parts, and the destructive remains of buildings symbolized for him the bad parts of himself which he found so hard to accept.

Regresssion

Regression was also an emphasis of Freud's early work as it helped to explain "fixations" as a cause of mental illness. Regression is going backward from a later to an earlier stage of development. In 1964, Arlow and Brenner defined regression as "the re-emergence of modes of mental functioning characteristic of earlier phases of psychic development." They further state that regressions are usually transient and reversible. Pathology is not determined by the depth of the regression (oral, anal, etc.) but by its irreversible nature, by the conflicts which it engenders and by its interference with the process of adaptation. The importance of regression has recently been enhanced by its relation to borderline and psychotic conditions. Psychotic individuals are said to be regressed to the oral stage (birth - 1 year), the earliest stage in Freud's psychosexual stages of development. Borderline (character disorder) individuals are thought to be regressed to the anal stage (1-3 years), and fixated there. This view of regression may help to explain the behavior of our patients with these diagnoses in terms of the functioning of the ego. To do so, however, would require a thorough understanding of Freud's psychosexual stages of development.

Regression has another implication that is important for the occupational therapist in planning treatment. This is the concept of "regression in the service of the ego." Ernst Kris (1936) first used this term to imply a purposeful regression to earlier modes of functioning without the loss of overriding ego control. The artist who smears paint on a canvas to express extreme affect but retains the control to return to the normal world (while the psychotic patient cannot) is a good example. The technique of "free association" or the uncensored, often illogical associations of words and images, has been cited as another example.

The therapeutic usefulness of regression to the ego lies in its contribution to a clearer self-understanding. When we ask our patients to wedge clay or use finger paints, these processes reflect the typical (sometimes forbidden) fascination of the anal stage (smearing feces). Our therapeutic purpose for doing this is not to encourage regression, but to free the individual to express affect in an uninhibited way, with the hope of recapturing the innate urge toward mastery which may be trapped there. The patient, after engaging in such a creative process, returns to a more mature level of functioning, but he retains an awareness of the affect discovered during the regression. This affect is essential if the patient is to change the way he understands and uses activity as a part of his return to healthy functioning.

Acting Out

Acting out can best be defined as an action, usually repetitive and compulsive in nature, and often self-destructive, that serves the unconscious purpose of resolving a repressed internal conflict by external means. This is a popular way to explain self-destructive behavior in analytical terms. It reflects a primitive lack of control over actions that are typical of the infant, and regressively present in psychosis and character disorder.

In groups, we often see emotions being "acted out" instead of talked about. For example, anger at someone in the group is expressed by walking out of the room and slamming the door. An action is substituted for a mature verbal description of a feeling state. Occupational therapist group leaders should discourage acting out responses. These are inappropriate and unproductive for both the patient and other group members. The more mature ego skill of verbal expression of affect should be encouraged.

Identification

Identification, as a defense described by Freud, was meant quite literally as the taking onto oneself the characteristics of another. The concept originated as a logical outcome of the Oedipal conflict, in which sexual desire for the opposite sex parent is replaced by identification with the parent of like sex. Anna Freud (1936) described this phenomenon as "identification with the aggressor." The child's identification with the feared "aggressor" is used, in part, to explain the repetition of behavior patterns in families. Child abuse is an example when the abused child grows up to abuse his own children. Erikson (1950) contributed greatly to the popularity of this concept in his extensive discussion of the identity crisis occurring in late adolescence.

Competence/Mastery

Bellak (1973) defines this function of the ego as adaptive performance in work and relationships, and the subjective feelings of competence. R.H. White defines competence as "an organism's capacity to interact effectively with it's environment..." (Bellak 1973, 260). "Fitness to interact with the environment" in White's view, includes language and motor skills, cognition and higher thought processes. The affect or feeling of efficacy is what White called "effectance motivation" (Bellak 1973, 260) referring to the individual's tendency to put more effort and energy into producing responses that will have a desirable effect on the environment. The feelings of competence are the result of a well-developed ego, and include a history of successful experiences in coping with the environment.

The ego's ability to cope is what rescues a person in times of illness or crisis. In an emotional crisis, many of the ego defenses described earlier may be viewed as coping mechanisms, protecting the ego from destruction by diverting psychic energy. In the case of physical trauma, the ego uses body sense and reality testing to determine what functions of the body remain intact. The ego's sense of self will often provide the motivation to find ways to compensate for lost functions. For example, a patient with right-sided hemiplegia will learn to write with his left hand. Compensation is a coping strategy.

Another example of a coping strategy is energy conservation. When physical and mental deterioration occur, energy for use in everyday activities is severely limited. Careful planning before embarking on a task can prevent the patient from wasting energy in needless movements. For example, after I had an operation, I was only able to stand up or walk for 15 minutes before stopping to take a rest. When preparing a meal, I had to learn to use the 15 minutes to gather absolutely everything I needed to make meatballs, then assemble them while sitting at the kitchen table. The cooking had to be done in an electric frying pan on the table, rather than at the stove. I had to learn to be satisfied with accumulating a mess around me, rather than cleaning as I went along, and to use a wet sponge to wipe my hands, rather than washing at the sink every few minutes. For patients with chronic disability, conserving energy is a coping skill that is absolutely essential for continued functioning at a level that is consistent with the patient's self-identity.

Function and Dysfunction

A functioning adult is free of conflicts and fixations, and is able to satisfy his or her needs and direct his or her drives in ways that fit in with the social environment and culture. A balance exists in the functioning individual that allows the psychic energy to flow freely between the id, ego and superego. The ego is in control and defense mechanisms are not exaggerated, so that the individual with a healthy ego can use most of his or her energy to grow and develop and interact effectively with others. In Fidler's model, the healthy person is able to work productively with others to accomplish a task. As an adult, he/she has acquired all six of Mosey's adaptive skills (Mosey 1981 - see Appendix A). The defenses the individual uses are mature ones, like sublimation of aggression in work, identification with idealized others and the suppression of immediate gratification. A healthy ego is synonymous with a strong sense of self; body image, self-identity and self-esteem are realistic, and can serve as the basis of adaptive function.

Dysfunction in the psychoanalytic frame of reference is defined in terms of inadequate psychosexual development, the presence of conflicts and fixations and the imbalance of psychic energy among the three parts of the personality. These abnormal states can produce symptoms of neurosis, psychosis or character disorder, which imply a disturbance in the ability to carry out activities of daily living.

Dysfunction can be seen as a lack of ego skills. This can take the form of poor reality testing, poor or unrealistic body image, poor self-identity, poor self-esteem, impulsiveness or passivity, unbalanced use of defenses and an inability to cope. Assessment of the ego functions will guide our setting of goals in occupational therapy. Patients with similar goals may be treated together in groups.

Change and Motivation

Change occurs through the learning and performance of adequate ego adaptive skills. These skills can be learned within the social context of therapeutic groups, where the consequences of problem behaviors can be readily seen and discussed. Foundation skills can be worked on through simple, well-structured, reality oriented tasks that focus on the development to sensory motor, perceptual and cognitive skills. Motivation can be enhanced through success experiences in occupational therapy.

Motivation comes from the directing of psychic energy toward the mastery of ego skills. When energy is bound up in dealing with conflict, persons may not be motivated to develop ego skills. As the ego is available to help reduce tensions and to satisfy needs through mature relationships and meaningful work activities, persons will be motivated to increase ego skill development. The occupational therapist can set up therapeutic groups that allow patients to practice adequate ego skills and experience successful and satisfying consequences for patients. A strong self-concept and high self-esteem are also motivating; these foster a sense of control and lead people to direct their energy toward even greater skill development.

Review of Occupational Therapy Perspective

The next portion of this chapter will review three authors from occupational therapy whose work has reflected the principles of the psychoanalytic frame of reference: Gail Fidler, Lela Llorens and Anne Mosey. Occupational therapy groups using this frame of reference became popular during the 1960s and '70s, and consequently many of the published works of these authors began about then.

An important influence in occupational therapy at the time of the early writings of Fidler, Llorens and Mosey was a treatment approach begun in England by Maxwell Jones (1953, 1968), known as the **therapeutic community**. The therapeutic community represented in the 1960s and '70s a fundamental change in approach to the treatment of mental illness. Both psychodynamic theories of personality and theories of sociology contributed to this unique approach, which called for the patient role to change from a "sick role" to that of a responsible community member. Hospitals and institutions all over Europe and America began therapeutic communities on their psychiatric units and occupational therapists were an integral part of this new approach.

Prior to the '60s, occupational therapy, although administered in groups, had a task skill focus with an emphasis on the use of crafts and productive work skills. The rise of therapeutic communities called for OTs to incorporate milieu principles into their treatment approach. Examples of these principles are 1) those most effected by a decision should be involved in making it (Jones 1953), 2)"in the context of responsibility for self and others, patients will alter their self perception from that of subordinate to that of peer group member" (Fairweather 1964), and 3) patients learn best when they are allowed to experience the consequences of their own actions.

The Task-Oriented Group—Fidler

In keeping with the times, Gail Fidler published her classic article, "The Task-Oriented Group as a Context for Treatment" in 1969 (Appendix A). She mentions several spokesmen for ego psychology in her rationale, such as Sullivan and Lewin, and points to the "emerging focus on ego functions and adaptive skills" (Fidler 1969, 43). Fidler also alludes to a focus on the use of groups in therapy, as "a dynamic force in facilitating learning and behavior change" (Lewin 1945).

Fidler, in incorporating occupational therapy principles with those of the therapeutic milieu, pointed out the value of observing patients doing tasks. She noted that "as patients engaged in activities or created objects, they expressed characterological difficulties, and that attention to these problems as they emerged and were operant in the here and now, seemed to be of benefit to the patient" (Fidler 1969, 45). There appeared to her to be a relationship between problems encountered by a patient in his activity experiences and those difficulties he encountered in the outside world. The assumption here is not unlike one made by the ego psychologists. If the patients' difficulties either interpersonally or in task performance are made conscious, whether by experience itself, group feedback or feedback from the therapist, the patient can utilize ego skills to cope with the difficulties. The strengthening of ego skills, then, becomes the goal of the task-oriented group.

Although the task is defined as either an end product or a service which is done by the group as a whole, Fidler points out that task accomplishment is not really the purpose. Rather, the task is intended to "provide a shared working experience wherein the relationship between feeling, thinking and behavior, their impact on others and on task accomplishment and productivity can be viewed and explored" (Fidler 1969, 45). Through the task group experience, ego skills and deficits can be observed in the patient. Patients demonstrate, in the process of participating in the group, their problems in interaction and in doing, and these problems can then be the focus of group problem-solving. Through both therapist and group feedback, "alternate patterns of functioning can be considered and tested within the context of the here and now, to the end that such learning may induce ego growth and improve function" (Fidler 1969, 45).

In other words, patients are expected to reflect on their behavior in the group and to come to some understanding of its consequence on other members and on task accomplishment. Behavior which is disturbing to others or counterproductive is identified as such, and presumably more adaptive modes of behavior are suggested and tried. The occupational therapist facilitates this process during the group; she intervenes as problems arise, points them out to the group and helps the group problem-solve. (See Appendix A for Fidler's article.)

Occupational Therapy in an Ego Adaptive Milieu–Llorens

Lela Llorens also wrote about occupational therapy programming using the psychoanalytic frame of reference. Her article, "Occupational therapy in an ego oriented milieu" with P. Johnson (1966) and her book, *Developing Ego Functions in Disturbed Children* with E. Rubin (1967), present useful occupational therapy assessment and treatment ideas using this practice model. Llorens writes that "a program of occupational therapy designed to enhance and support adaptive functioning must provide for the development of ego skills, opportunities for practice and support for mastery" (1966, 179). She describes occupational therapy groups in three phases of treatment: evaluation, convalescence and rehabilitation.

In the **evaluation** phase, observation is emphasized. The group meets three consecutive days for one hour each day, and activities include orientation to occupational therapy, written completion of a background information sheet and completion of a small mosaic tile tray. This small sample of behavior allows the occupational therapist to observe the patient's mood, relationships, motivation, performance and skills. Results of the evaluation show how well the patient's ego is functioning in helping him/her adapt to the environment. Those whose egos are functioning less than normal are assigned to the convalescent phase of treatment.

The goals of the **convalescent** phase are to promote increased feelings of adequacy and to encourage independence in functioning. Modalities suggested to achieve these goals are sewing and needlework, art, leather and metal work and woodwork. Convalescent groups consist of five to fifteen patients with two therapists. Some ego skills worked on in this phase are 1) expression or sublimation of needs in an acceptable manner, 2) attention span and work tolerance, 3) reality testing and orientation and 4) verbal and non-verbal communication of feelings. The therapist takes responsibility for planning in these groups according to the patient's ability.

Patients whose egos are more highly functional are placed in the **rehabilitation** phase of occupational therapy treatment. Modalities for groups in this phase include more interaction: male and female interest groups, activities of daily living discussion group, graceful living, typing and cooking. A less authoritative leadership style is used in these groups. Mastery is both the motivation and the goal.

Adaptive Skills and Developmental Groups–Mosey

Anne Cronin Mosey's concept of adaptive skills is also useful in the psychoanalytic frame of reference. While she frames the adaptive skills in a developmental context, (recapitulation of ontogenesis), the skills themselves closely resemble many of the functions of the ego described earlier. According to Mosey, "the term adaptive is used to indicate that these skills are acquired and utilized by the individual so that he may satisfy his inherent needs and the needs of others, interact with the environment in order to attain personal goals, and knowledgeably select those environmental demands he wishes to meet" (1970, 134). Mosey acknowledges the influence of psychoanalytic theory on the adaptive skills by accepting the concepts of conscious, preconscious, unconscious, complex formation and regression, but adds the need for mastery as an important component. She proposes that fixation may be the result of deficient adaptive skill learning. She identifies six adaptive skills, which are learned in sequence, with some overlap and interdependence as the child matures: 1) perceptual-motor skill, 2) cognitive skill, 3) dyadic interaction skill, 4) group interaction skill, 5) self-identity skill and 6) sexual identity skill. The idea that group interaction skill precedes and therefore needs to be mastered *before* self-identity or gender identity are possible is significant. For an elaboration on these, the reader is referred to Mosey's book, *Psychosocial Components of Occupational Therapy* (1986). (See Appendix C for a complete list of Mosey's adaptive skills and subskills.)

Summary of Mosey's Developmental Groups

Of particular interest to occupational therapists working with groups are the components of group interaction skill described by Mosey. She suggests five types of non-familial groups which simulate those which may be encountered in normal development. The intention of these groups is to provide opportunities to develop group interaction skills in the correct developmental sequence. Group interaction skill is "the ability to participate in a variety of groups in a manner that is satisfying for oneself and for one's fellow group members" (Mosey 1970 *AJOT*, 273). The five types of groups are 1) parallel,

2) project, 3) egocentric-cooperative, 4) cooperative and 5) mature (Mosey 1986). (See Appendix B for Mosey's article describing these groups.)

Parallel Groups

Parallel groups are the lowest level, made up of patients doing individual tasks side by side. Preschool children may be observed in a similar process on a playground, one swinging, another climbing, another digging in the sandbox. Little interaction is required, and the therapist defines the task and provides patients with the necessary assistance and emotional support.

Project Groups

Project groups emphasize task accomplishment. Some interaction may be built-in, such as shared materials and tools and sharing the work. Social interaction outside of the task is not expected. The therapist structures the group with tasks that require interaction of two or more persons to complete.

Egocentric-Cooperative Groups

Egocentric-cooperative groups require the members to select and implement the task. Tasks are longer term and social interaction is expected. Although the task serves to organize this group, members are expected to respond to one another's social and emotional needs. The therapist facilitates this process.

Cooperative Groups

Cooperative groups require the therapist only as an advisor. Members are "encouraged to identify and gratify each other's social and emotional needs in conjunction with task accomplishment" (Mosey 1970, 273). The task in the cooperative group may be secondary to social aspects.

Mature Groups

In mature groups, the therapist is a co-equal member. The group members take on all the necessary leadership roles in order to balance task accomplishment with need satisfaction of the members.

Group Treatment

Occupational therapy writers have implied that ego functions can be both evaluated and developed (learned) in the context of task-focused groups. The task, in groups using a psychoanalytic frame, takes on greater importance than in humanistic groups. Even when the task is not the focus, it is the *context* in which discussion, problem-solving and therapeutic change take place. Therefore the structure of the occupational therapy group in this frame is fundamentally different.

Structure and Limitations

After the introduction, the task predominates the group session providing both the structure and the time frame for the group. Tasks can last for part of one session, or go on for several sessions. A task might take three hours at one time. Discussion depends on problems that arise and how the therapist chooses to intervene. Evaluative discussion is left for the last fifteen minutes of each session, with a longer evaluation reserved following the end of the task. This alternative structure is primarily based on Fidler's "task-oriented group" but has been expanded and further defined. Mosey's concept of developmental groups is reflected in the changing role of the leader. The leader gives more help and structure to groups that are less capable, and less help to groups that have a higher level of ego functioning. The task group is not limited to high functioning patients. It can be adapted to fairly low levels of group interaction skill, with some changes in structure and the amount of help given by the leader.

Role of the Leader

Fidler defines the role of the occupational therapist as one of a facilitator. The leader's major goal is to make learning possible, and not to take over the group. Facilitation, then, requires that the therapist maintain and communicate a basic belief in the group's capacity to be "constructively self-determining" (Fidler 1969, 46). This means she does not make decisions for the group, or rescue the group from its difficulties. Rather, she intervenes in the group's process in ways that encourage the group to make its own decisions and solve its own problems. The therapist decides how much freedom she will allow the group to be self-determining, based on her assessment of the level of ego functioning of group members. There is a delicate balance between success and failure and she should not permit the group to become immobilized with frustration when it is truly incapable of doing a task or solving a problem without her help. This kind of leadership requires a thorough understanding of group dynamics.

Goals

The goals of groups in the psychoanalytic frame are for patients to develop and practice ego skills. These skills, reviewed from the beginning of the chapter, are reality testing, body image, self-identity, self-esteem, sense of control and the use of healthy defenses and coping strategies. Providing the foundation for these skills are cognitive, perceptual and sensorimotor skills. Patients can be encouraged to develop and practice these skills within the group context through the shared working experience of tasks.

Examples of Activities

The group itself should decide on the task, using the resources of its members. Some of the successful task groups are reviewed here. Most tasks offer many opportunities to develop and reinforce ego skills. A few of these are highlighted for each group, but it is likely that many others are also possible.

A Group Newspaper

The group consisted of six Vietnam veterans who exhibited symptoms of substance abuse and post traumatic stress syndrome. This was significant in their choice of a task. They decided that what was most meaningful to them was to "tell the world the truth" about Vietnam veterans. The group took a trip to the library, where books and articles on the Vietnam war and on Post Traumatic Stress Syndrome were read and notes taken. From the notes, articles were written. Group members added their own stories, poems and drawings, as well as old newspaper articles they had saved. The result was a twenty-page booklet that was typed, copied, collated and widely distributed to veterans hospital patients and staff by the group members.

In this group, members' common self-identity as "the unsung heros" was reinforced. The task facilitated a sense of control by giving members a vehicle for expression of feelings and opinions that was acceptable in the social environment. Self-esteem was increased by the recognition of their work by others.

Easter Chocolates

The chocolates were really a combination of a product and service project. The group knew of a local residential school for handicapped children, and wanted to do something for them. Since Easter was the next holiday, they decided to give them Easter candy. But they were on a limited budget, so they came up with the idea of making candy instead of buying it. Candy molds, baker's chocolate, sugar and tin foil were the only purchases. Members were able to collect enough old Easter baskets to hold the wrapped candy. The candy was made in the shapes of eggs, chicks and small bunnies. Members wrapped each piece in foil and placed them in the baskets. Two of the group members delivered the baskets to the staff of the residential school the week before Easter. A week later they were very proud to receive a big thank-you letter from the children.

Self-identity and esteem were reinforced in this group through doing for others. Members learned that they were capable of producing a product that brought pleasure to others, and were recognized for their altruism. Identification as a healthy defense was encouraged through nurturing the children (by giving candy) as perhaps they might have wished to be nurtured themselves.

A Walk to the Pet Store

The most important factor to this group was to get away from the hospital. They were psychiatric patients and not even allowed to walk around the grounds unescorted. In the task group, walking to the pet store gave them a way to go out as a group during scheduled group time, escorted by the occupational therapy staff. They decided on the destination because it was only a fifteen minute walk, it was always interesting to see and it wouldn't cost any money. This task group gave them the opportunity to plan something together to meet their needs, restoring in them some sense of control. The sensory stimulation of walking and being in the outdoor environment also increased sensory motor skills.

Cooking a Spaghetti Dinner

Almost every group seems to enjoy a cooking task. It's relatively short term, provides enough work for all the members to participate and satisfies a basic need for everyone, the need to eat. If possible, the group can do the menu planning and shopping, as well as the actual meal preparation. Since spaghetti and salad can feed the whole group for relatively little money, the group was able to afford soft drinks and dessert as well. This group made brownies from a mix before beginning the main course. Members were divided into salad makers, spaghetti makers, dessert makers and table setters. The meal was enjoyed by the whole group and everyone was expected to help clean up.

This group requires many adaptive ego functions. Members identify with different roles to work on a realistic goal. They use their skills to cope with their part of the task, and receive feedback from others about their performance (reality testing). All of the senses are stimulated through the cooking task, and impulse control is necessary when using the tools and equipment (knives, stove).

Group Car Wash

This task required the cooperation of the hospital or sponsoring institution to provide permission, a space to work and a source of water. At the VA Hospital, the group took on the responsibility of writing letters to the various hospital administrators asking for permission. The letters were followed up with phone calls from the occupational therapist and other staff. Supplies included buckets, soap, rags, sponges and a nozzle for the hose, most of which were borrowed from relatives and friends. Members prepared for the car wash one week ahead by making signs to post all over the hospital. On the day of the car wash a few group members, accompanied by staff, went outside to post signs and arrows on the street and in the parking lot directing customers to the car wash location. Patients and staff took shifts of two hours each for six hours. At $3 a car, the group made almost $200, which they spent on a video tape player so the whole ward could watch movies on weekends.

Patience and perseverence were required in the planning of this extended task. There were many opportunities to reality test, reinforce body image (gross motor actions), self-identity (through working roles) and self-esteem (through the concrete result of their effort).

Group Leadership

In this frame of reference, as suggested earlier, the structure of the group is modified to include most of the discussion areas in the context of the activity or task. The activity, sharing, processing, generalizing and application are not done as separate phases of the group, but are incorporated into the process of doing the task. Since the goal is to develop ego skills, the leader may stop the group whenever an opportunity for members to learn becomes evident. The evaluation portion should include all of the discussion phases of the group and should end with a summary.

Introduction

This part of the group can dispense with the warm-up and replace it with choosing a task. In beginning a task-oriented group, it is helpful for the leader to set forth some ground rules. Some of these will be specific, such as when and where the group will meet, for how long, and the practical limitations to their choice of task, such as availability of supplies. The leader also needs to set forth the expectation that the group will choose a task that they can all work on together, and that once decided, every member of the group is expected to contribute to task accomplishment. Three phases of a task group are introduced: 1) planning, 2) doing and 3) evaluating. The time frame may vary according to the task, and a thorough discussion will be delayed until the task itself is finished.

Phase 1 - Planning

After a brief introduction by the facilitator, the planning phase begins with brainstorming.

Brainstorming

Brainstorming involves the suggestion of possible tasks for the group by all members. Cooking a meal, planning a group walk, learning to do needlepoint and making Easter baskets for the pediatrics ward are some examples of group tasks. It is often useful for a member of the group to record the ideas. The therapist should caution the group not to make judgments of the ideas suggested during brainstorming, but just to collect a list of ideas.

Persuasion

The next step in planning is **persuasion**. Members consider the pros and cons of each suggestion and attempt to persuade the group to do one of them. Here the therapist may need to introduce the idea of meaningfulness. A task which is likely to succeed is one that has meaning for its members. It is very tempting for some groups to plan something easy to accomplish, but often the easy tasks hold little value for the members. This results in member residence in the doing phase. While the therapist should not under any circumstance influence the decision of the group, she should perhaps point out that a better decision will be made when the opinions of every member have been voiced and considered.

Interventions of the leader should be carefully thought out so as not to exert more authority than is necessary. Groups with poor ego skills will need more help than those with stronger ego skills. When in doubt, it is best to allow the group to experience the consequences of its actions, and then to find something to be learned from whatever happens. Occupational therapists often have difficulty with allowing groups to "fail" or to turn out badly. In the task-oriented group, however, it is often from the "failures" that patients can learn the most. Successful groups are of benefit in many ways also, but it is often the failures that promote real therapeutic change.

For example, I have sometimes observed in task-oriented groups with members of varied diagnoses, ages and functioning levels, an inability to make a group decision, even after 45 or 50 minutes of group discussion. Nothing is more frustrating to a group than sitting and doing nothing for an hour because nothing was planned. It is a mistake groups usually don't make twice. The planning session following such a group usually turns out to be quite productive.

Decision

After more or less persuasion, the group is expected to reach some kind of decision. Group decisions are made in several ways. Someone in the group can take a vote, with the majority ruling. Perhaps a consensus will be reached on the last suggestion discussed; if no one voices an objection, it may be assumed that everyone agrees. A patient leader might emerge in the group whose preference might be deferred to by the other members, or a decision can be made by a process of elimination. However the decision is made, it must be considered at some point during planning to be final. Often the group needs for the decision to be acknowledged and approved by the leader in order to proceed.

Specific Planning and Division of Labor

Once a decision is made, how the task will be accomplished should become the topic of discussion. Questions about what equipment and supplies are needed, how these will be obtained, where the group should be held and how necessary procedures will be learned are addressed. The facilitator, in this phase, often needs to be a resource to the group, offering his/her knowledge of supply sources, procedures and space availability. In lower functioning groups, this information should be offered more readily; in higher functioning groups, the therapist may offer information only if asked. The discussion of procedures naturally leads to the division of labor (who will do what). It is best when all the planning and preparation can be done by group members. Often each patient is charged with the responsibility of obtaining some item and bringing it to the group. Each member bringing one ingredient for a fruit salad or a pizza is an example of this. In this way it is easily seen that the success of the group task is dependent on each member of the group remembering and carrying out his or her responsibility.

Phase 2 - Doing

It is usually most practical for the doing phase to be done at least a day or two later than the planning. This gives members a chance to prepare adequately. On the day of the activity, **gathering** and **organizing** is best left up to group members, although they may need some help. If moving right into **activity** is something that works for the group, then the leader should allow this. Generally, if careful planning has been done, then not a great deal of time is needed to organize the doing. As members proceed with doing the activity, the facilitator's role may expand to include consulting, advising and providing information. The leader should be careful to offer these services only when asked, or when group disorganization is imminent. It is the role of the facilitator, however, to look for problems, and to bring these to the attention of the group along the way. As problems arise, the leader may apprise the group: "Mary seems to be feeling left out." or "Sam seems to be doing all the work." Care should be taken *not* to suggest solutions until it is evident that the group cannot cope with the problem on its own.

Phase 3 - Evaluation

Doing is not complete until the task is finished. However, evaluation of the group should be done before the end of every session. Sessions should be sufficiently long to allow for this process to occur. It is usually necessary for the leader to let the group know when it's time to stop doing and start talking. Discussion should focus on the process of the group and the role each member has chosen to play. The discussion phases of processing, generalizing and application are incorporated into this evaluation phase of task groups.

Reflection of Behavior and its Consequences

This should be verbalized if members are to learn from their experiences. Why was Mary feeling left out? Did she withdraw because she is shy? Was she seeking attention through non-participation? Was she uncertain about how to do her part of the task? Was she threatened by the perceived dominance of another member? How well did the group cope with Mary's problem? How did Mary feel? How did others feel about her? What other choices did the group have regarding Mary? These are the types of issues that should arise in evaluation of the group.

Feelings of Members About the Group

This "processing" aspect is an important part of evaluation. If Sam feels really good about the group, but Mary feels terrible, what are the reasons for this? Could Sam be feeling good because he's doing the whole thing himself and not allowing Mary an opportunity to contribute? How do other members see this? Suppose most of the members are bored with the task? What do they think makes it boring? How are they responsible for the boredom? What can they do about it? A leader should be very reluctant to allow a group to abandon a task part way through. Opportunities to learn should determine what is to be gained or lost from the abandonment. Most of the time the group can learn more from following through on a task, even if to do so is frustrating and problematic. However, if the group is overwhelmed by frustration, the members' anxiety may interfere with their ability to learn. This is another judgment call which may be difficult for the leader to make.

Evaluation of Task Accomplishment

Finally, an overall evaluation of task accomplishment is in order. How does the group feel about the result? How does it compare with what they hoped for/expected? What did each member contribute to its accomplishment? To what extent did planning affect outcome? It is in this phase that the relationship between thinking, feeling and behavior is most evident, and the therapist should never miss an opportunity to emphasize it. Good planning (thinking) generally produces successful action (behavior) and results in good feelings about oneself and the group. Concurrently, bad planning often produces an unsuccessful outcome and promotes bad feelings about self and the group. Individual examples of this process might also be pointed out. In all cases, learning from mistakes should be emphasized, so that members develop the strength and skill for making things turn out better next time.

Task-oriented groups are an excellent example of occupational therapy treatment using the psychoanalytic frame of reference. It is a context in which all of the ego skills discussed can be evaluated and worked on. However, it should be noted that it is not the only approach that works in this frame. Groups which use the symbolic meaning of activities or encourage self-expression through art, poetry, drama, dance/movement or creative writing are alternative group goals. Occupational therapy groups that encourage exploring the unconscious and uncovering painful or conflictual memories to be resolved remain a less popular, but an equally legitimate, application of psychoanalytic theory.

Bibliography

Allport G. *Becoming: Basic Considerations For a Psychology of Personality*. New Haven: Yale Univ. Press, 1958.
Arlow and Brenner. *Psychoanalytic Concepts and the Structural Theory*. New York: Int. Univ. Press, 1964.
Bellak L., Huruich M., Gediman H. *Ego Functions in Schizophrenics, Neurotics and Normals*. NY: Wiley & Sons, 1973.
Bergman M. and Hartman F. *The Evolution of Psychoanalytic Technique*. NY: Basic Books, 1976.
Bruce M. and Borg B. *Frames of Reference in Psychosocial Occupational Therapy*. NJ: SLACK Incorporated, 1987.
Corey G. *Theory and Practice of Counseling and Psychotherapy*. 4th ed. Monterey, CA: Brooks/Cole, 1991.
Diasio K. Psychiatric occupational therapy: Search for a conceptual framework in light of psychoanalytic ego psychology and learning theory. *AJOT*, 1968, XXII, 5, 50-57.
Erikson E. *Childhood and Society*, NY: Norton, 1950.
Fairweather G.W. *Social Psychology in Treating Mental Illness*. NY: Wiley & Sons, 1964.
Fidler G. *Design of Rehabilitation Services in Psychiatric Hospital Settings*. Laurel, MD: Ramsco, 1984.
Fidler G. The task-oriented group as a context for treatment.*AJOT*, 1969, XXIII, 1, 43-48.
Fine R. *A History of Psychoanalysis*. NY: Columbia University Press, 1979.
Freud A. *The Ego and the Mechanisms of Defense*. NY: Intl. University Press, 1936.
Freud S. History of the psychoanalytic movement. (In Strachey J. (19-14) *The Standard Edition of the Complete Psychological Works of Sigmund Freud*. London: Hogarth, 1914. (All other S. Freud references are from this text also.)
Greene L. and Cole M. Level and form of psychopathology and the structure of group therapy. *Int J Group Psychotherapy*, 1991.

Hartmann H. *Ego Psychology and the Problem of Adaptation*. NY: Intl. Univ. Press, 1939.

Jung C. The association method. *Am J of Psychology*, 1910, 21,216-269.

Kaplan H. and Sadock B. *Synopsis of Psychiatry*. 5th ed. Baltimore: Williams & Wilkins, 1988.

Kernberg O. Psychoanalytic studies of group processes: Theory and applications. (In Grinspoon L (Ed.), *Psychiatry Update*, 1983, Vol II (pp21-35). Washington DC: American Psychiatric Press).

Klein M. *Contributions to Psychoanalysis 1921-1945*. London: Hogarth Press, 1948.

Kris E. The Psychology of Characterature, *IJP*, 1936, 17, 285-303.

Llorens L. Occupational therapy in an ego-oriented milieu. *AJOT* 1966, XX, 4, 178-181.

Llorens L. and Rubin E. *Developing Ego Functions in Disturbed Children*. Detroit: Wayne State Univ. Press, 1967.

Llorens L. *Application of a Developmental Theory for Health and Rehabilitation*. Rockville, MD: American Occupational Therapy Association, 1976.

Mosey A. *Three Frames of Reference for Mental Health*. Thorofare, NJ: SLACK Inc., 1970.

Mosey A. The concept and use of developmental groups. *AJOT*, 1970, XXIV, 4, 272-275.

Mosey A. *Psychosocial Components of Occupational Therapy*. NY: Raven Press, 1986.

Mosey A. The Proper Focus of Scientific Inquiry in Occupational Therapy: Frames of Reference. *OTJR*, 1989, 9, 4, 195-201.

Murray. Uses of the thematic apperception test. *Am. J of Psychiatry*, 1951, 107, 577-81.

Rapaport D. *Emotions and Memory*. NY: Harper, 1942.

Rapaport D. On the psychoanalytic theory of affects. *IJP*, 1953, 34, 177-198.

Rorshach. *Psychodiagnostics: A Diagnostic Test Based on Perception*. NY: Grune & Stratton, 1921.

Spitz R. *A Genetic Field Theory Ego Formation: It's Implications for Pathology*. NY: Intl. U. Press, 1959.

Wechsler D. *Wechsler Adult Intelligence Scale*. Rev. ed. NY: The Psychological Corporation, 1981.

Witkin H. et.al. *Personality Through Perception*. NY: Harper, 1954.

Chapter

5

Cognitive Approaches

The first approach discussed here is the cognitive disabilities theory of Claudia Allen. Allen's basic premise is that behavior is based on cognition, and in order to produce change in behavior, the thinking process must change. Many of the patients we will treat in occupational therapy are cognitively impaired. Allen has organized a heirarchy of six cognitive levels and described typical behaviors of each. Using her guidelines, we can easily evaluate our patients and place them in activity groups that are appropriate for their cognitive level. However, because we see a broad range of cognitive abilities in acute care settings, a broad range of techniques is required. Because more learning is possible at Allen's levels 5 and 6 (highest), patients at these levels can benefit from occupational therapy approaches based on the concepts of cognitive behaviorism (Allen, November 17, 1992, personal communication).

Therefore, the second set of concepts discussed in this chapter is cognitive behaviorism. Cognitive behaviorism is one of the most frequently used in psychiatry for several reasons. It sounds simple and logical, it easily lends itself to advances in technology, such as computer programing and biofeedback, and it is appropriate and useful in short term treatment. Occupational therapists use the concepts from cognitive behaviorism in treating patients on a verbal and symbolic level. To benefit from this approach, it is suggested that patients be at least an Allen's level 5 or 6, capable of learning through logic and reasoning. The principal spokesmen for the cognitive behavioral therapies in psychology are identified by Bruce and Borg (1987) as Albert Bandura, Aaron Beck and Albert Ellis. Both Allen and the cognitive behaviorists share the guiding principle that therapy should focus on the cognitive process, and that it is changes in thinking that will produce adaptive changes in patient behavior.

In combining these theoretical approaches, I have spoken extensively with Claudia Allen, and we have agreed that many occupational therapists are misinformed about how cognitive disabilities theory relates to cognitive behaviorism. In this chapter, I hope to clarify this relationship. In occupational therapy, they can be seen as a part of the same continuum. Allen draws on some of the same theoretical concepts, but applies them to task performance in persons with cognitive limitations (Allen Dec. 28, 1991, personal communication).

Basic Assumptions

From a historical perspective, behaviorism is an extreme stance which developed in the 1940's and 1950's in direct opposition to psychoanalytic theory. Like Freudian id psychology, behaviorism is deterministic in that it rejects the notion that human beings are free agents who decide on their own destiny. But Freud believed that personality is shaped by internal biological forces, while behaviorists contend that behavior and personality are determined by past and present events in the external world. Behaviorists were the first to apply a scientific experimental method to the study of human behavior.

Just as ego psychology was an outgrowth of psychoanalytic theory, cognitive behaviorism has advanced from the original behavioral theories. Cognitive behaviorists basically accept the principles of behavior modification, but have added thinking to the repertoire of human behavior that can be learned and modified. The fundamental change these psychological theories have made from their predecessors is their rejection of determinism. Just as the concept of ego autonomy implies that man can adapt and change according to his own will, cognition in the cognitive frame allows man to regulate his own behavior. This concept has important implications for treatment.

Allen—Cognitive Disabilities Theory

Claudia Allen has been developing the theory of cognitive disabilities since the late 1960's. She estimates about 80% of the patients we treat in occupational therapy have some form of cognitive disability. Allen's concept of change may not fit with the theories of the cognitive behaviorists, but her contention that cognition is a central determinant of behavior is similar. Allen's contributions are based on a rehabilitation view of change that involves living with the consequences of health problems.

Allen accepts the concept that a person's cognitive level has biological and chemical determinants. Treatment may or may not eliminate the disorder. If eliminated, the therapist verifies the absence of a functional disability. If not eliminated, the therapist assists the patient and other caregivers in making the necessary adjustments required by a residual cognitive disability. Claudia Allen does a great deal to operationalize the theories of cognitive behaviorism in the occupational therapy clinic. However, she does not label her work as cognitive behavioral "because she perceives an element of free choice operating in all conscious, living organisms" (Allen 1991, personal communication).

Six Cognitive Levels

First, Allen divides cognitive disabilities into six well-defined cognitive levels, and provides several assessment tools to help OTs evaluate the cognitive level. Assessment and treatment are based on how the patient learns and performs tasks. The cognitive levels are largely presented as descriptions of typical behaviors at that level. A summary of the levels follows. For a more complete understanding of these levels and their assessment, the reader is referred to Allen's books (Allen 1985, Allen and Earhart 1992).

Level 1 - Automatic Actions

The level 1 patient is in most cases bedridden. He/she is conscious but responds mainly to internal or subliminal cues (sensations from within the body). Behavior is largely habitual or reflexive. Arousal and response to others may be elicited for a few seconds at a time. Most daily needs (dressing, grooming, feeding) have to be done by caretakers.

Level 2 - Postural Actions

At level 2, patients can be stimulated to perform postural actions (changes in position) in response to proprioceptive (sense of motion and position) cues. Patients can imitate gross motor actions, and can assist a caregiver in bathing, dressing and grooming. Usually level 2 patients can feed themselves, although this may be messy. Twenty-four hour nursing care is required.

Level 3 - Manual Actions

At this level patients perform manual actions (movements with their hands) in response to tactile cues (touch). Actions based on interest in objects found within hand's reach may be repeated many times. Attention can be maintained up to thirty minutes. Basic daily grooming tasks may be done independently with reminders: patients can walk to familiar places but get easily lost in new surroundings. Repetitive work tasks can be done at level three. Some of the tasks requiring supervision are care of belongings and clothing, money management, preparing meals, following a schedule and use of a telephone.

Level 4 - Goal-Directed Actions

Level 4 patients perform goal-directed actions in response to visual cues. These patients are able to complete short tasks such as making a sandwich or washing the dishes. Attention is up to one hour and steps toward a goal can be imitated one at a time. Patients perform most daily self care activities but need assistance in coping with new events, anticipating needs, and managing money. Visual stimuli are the focus, and non-visible safety hazards (a hot stove, for example) may be a danger. Directions for getting places or doing tasks must be demonstrated visually, since verbal and written directions are not followed.

Level 5 - Exploratory Actions

Use of trial and error is the hallmark of level 5. Persons use inductive reasoning and are capable of new learning. Basic living skills are intact: grooming, dressing, toileting, bathing and feeding. Patients at level 5 can imitate new procedures and remember several steps at a time. In task performance, novelty is sought and variation explored.

Deficits at level five are in functions that require anticipation and planning. These are concrete thinkers primarily, and have trouble imagining the long-term consequences of their actions or inactions. Hence, preventative measures are often not taken. In the home, for example, needed repairs may be neglected (a broken step is neglected until someone trips and falls). Cooking presents a problem when timing is involved: burning is not anticipated, for example. Money management is a major problem since level five patients seldom save for emergencies or anticipate future expenses. Also neglected are purchasing needed items for a meal, cleaning or laundering clothing and getting prescriptions refilled. The lack of abstract thinking prevents these patients from understanding the nature of their illness or the effects of medication. Jobs and social relationships may suffer because of failure to anticipate the consequences of self-centered behavior.

Level 6 - Planned Actions

This is the highest level and represents the absence of disability. The main distinguishing characteristic is the ability to use deductive reasoning and to plan ahead. Future events are anticipated and behavior is organized. Verbal and written directions can be followed without demonstration and the person is able to use symbolic cues (Allen 1988).

Cognitive Disability Group Treatment

Treatment group membership in occupational therapy is based on cognitive level. Patients are treated in homogeneous groups of similar cognitive level. Level 2 is the lowest that can be treated effectively within a group. Earhart (in Allen 1985) suggests that in a large facility a variety of groups should be offered for levels 2-6. Some patients will move up a level or two as their acute symptoms remit. Others will stabilize at a lower level and will require a variety of tasks within that level. Activities appropriate for each level are suggested. Table 5-1 describing the cognitive abilities of patients at each of the six levels can serve as a guide for planning activities. The table is based on an earlier chart by Allen, revised by Mary Brinson and Mary Ann Mayer.

Level 2 Groups

Movement activities are suggested to meet the needs of the level 2 patients (level 3 patients may also be included). Activities consist of imitation of gross body movement such as clapping, bending over to touch toes and passing or tossing a large, soft ball may be useful, although a level 2 patient is apt to disregard directionality. The disruptive behavior of level 2 or 3 patients in groups is oblivious to verbal direction but often responsive to demonstrated direction.

Level 3 and 4 Groups

For level 3 and 4 groups, Earhart (in Allen 1985) suggests several activities: basic grooming, basic crafts, basic sewing and basic skills. Since vision is central at level 4, the tasks should be shown in pictures or samples and suggested by the materials laid out. A grooming group, for example, may be given the choice of doing fingernails, toenails, hair or shave their face or legs. Materials for these tasks should be set out for patients to see. However, level 3 patients are distracted by too many materials, and for them only the necessary items for doing a chosen task should remain visible. Level 3 and 4 patients are not able to find supplies or anticipate the need for preparation. Level 3 patients will perform repetitive actions such as filing nails and combing hair, while level 4's prefer to see a finished sample such as a picture or nail filed by the therapist. Familiar tasks are best at these lower cognitive levels.

Another suggested group for levels 3 and 4 is basic crafts. This group is popular among psychiatric and geriatric patients. Up to ten patients can be treated by one therapist when the task environment minimizes distraction. Patients sit at tables and work side by side for up to one hour. Projects are designed to be completed in one session. Preparation is critical - tasks should be analyzed to include visual and manual action components while avoiding non-visible procedures or the use of other than simple tools. For craft projects, a completed sample is necessary for demonstration. Materials for the project are set up ahead of time by the therapist. Everything must be ready to use, paints opened and

Table 5-1.
Task Analysis for Cognitive Disabilities

	LEVEL 1: Automatic Actions	LEVEL 2: Postural Actions	LEVEL 3: Manual Actions
Setting	Reduce the number of stimuli when possible. Patients do not screen out external stimuli.	Open space. Patients enjoy planned gross motor actions.	Clutter free. Patients are engaged in doing simple tasks which have repetitive actions.
THE THERAPIST'S DIRECTIONS			
Demonstrations	Looks at demonstrated directions but does not imitate them.	The therapist may need to physically guide the action.	Patients will follow a demonstration of a familiar action on an object.
Verbalizations	Verbs, introjections.	Pronouns, names of body parts, simple verbs reinforce demonstration.	Names of material objects, repeated simple nouns and verbs.
Number of Directions	One action or direction, repeated	One action or direction, repeated	One action or direction, repeated
TASK SELECTION			
Structure of the Activity	Alerting stimuli. The most important tasks are eating and drinking.	Familiar, repetitive gross body movements.	An activity which has one step or one scheme repeated.
Choice and Sample Provided		The therapist plans movements and demonstrates actions. The therapist may respond to patient's suggestions or actions.	Activity is pre-planned by therapist. Choices limited to two or three material items/objects.
Tools	Stimulated use of body parts	Spontaneous use of body parts. Objects which are associated with gross body movements eg, softballs, jump ropes.	Hands: Some use of familiar tools.
Storage of Materials/ Projects	Taken care of by the therapist.	Taken care of by the therapist.	Taken care of by the therapist.
Preparation by the Therapist		Plan movements and obtain any needed equipment.	Supplies are laid out in advance. Do any preliminary or finishing steps which are not repetitive or familiar.

Copyright Mary Ann Mayer and Mary H. Brinson; information gathered from Allen (1987) Cognitive Disabilities: Measuring Social Consequences of mental disorders, JClin Psychiatry, 48, 181-191.

stirred, sandpaper right side up, protective newspaper covering the table. Clutter is very distracting. Only materials needed for the current step of the project should be presented. The therapist must demonstrate each step to the entire group as well as giving simple verbal directions. Basic sewing, most preferable to female patients, is set up to run in a similar fashion.

Basic skills, a group intended for level 4, uses an educational approach to teach community survival skills. Since new learning is not possible at level 4, the purpose is to review what living skills patients already know and to reinforce their use. Examples of

Table 5-1. (Continued)
Task Analysis for Cognitive Disabilities

	LEVEL 4: Goal-directed Actions	LEVEL 5: Exploratory Actions	LEVEL 6: Planned Actions
Setting	Other patients working on the same task, a shared goal. Setting conducive to production of immediate end product.	Clutter can be present, and others performing variations on similar tasks. Setting fosters exploration, trial and error.	Free access to materials and supplies to stimulate covert problem-solving, sharing of plans with others.
THE THERAPIST'S DIRECTIONS			
Demonstrations	Patients will imitate single steps in a series and moderately novel actions which expand familiar schemes.	Patients can learn through serial imitation, so a number of steps may be demonstrated. Unfamiliar steps assimiliated.	Not required. Patients learn through serial imitations so directions may be retained.
Verbalizations	Simple adjectives, adverbs nouns and verbs; avoiding open-ended questions or discussions.	Adjectives and prepositions may be used in explaining variations.	Conjunctions, conjectures, images.
Number of Directions	One step at a time.	Several steps at a time.	Unlimited. Images, diagrams, written directions may be followed.
TASK SELECTION			
Structure of the Activity	Simple quick tasks with a tangible end product. Avoid childish connotations.	An activity which permits variation, and which allows results to be easily seen and corrected.	An activity which permits variation in the selection and planning of steps.
Choice and Sample Provided	Avoid confusion by limiting the decisions and materials. The opportunity for exact replication of a sample is present.	Several choices in materials, tools and activity selection. Demonstrate and clarify tangible possibilities.	Several choices in materials, tools, and activity selection. Discuss the hypothetical possibilities.
Tools	Hand tools limited to familiar objects. No power tools.	Simple tools which are a linear extension of the hand and arm.	Patients learn how to use unfamiliar machines and tools.
Storage of Materials/ Projects	Patients will place and/or find supplies when clearly visible or very familiar.	The patient will search for things in probable locations and can place/ find things in labeled drawers or cabinets.	The patient will follow verbal directions to place or find materials
Preparation by the Therapist	Supplies are laid out in advance. Provide an exact sample of the end product. Do those steps which require unfamiliar tools or schemes.	The sample of the finished product need not be exact. Patterns and procedures are supplied by the therapist.	Materials, designs, and/or pictures are provided to assist covert problem-solving.

Copyright Mary Ann Mayer and Mary H. Brinson; information gathered from Allen (1987) Cognitive Disabilities: Measuring Social Consequences of mental disorders, *JClin Psychiatry*, 48, 181-191.

activities are doing laundry, reading directions for taking prescription medication, making change from a purchase, taking a bus, ordering from a restaurant menu, and using a telephone directory. Some exercises are designed to renew intellectual skills, such as vocabulary review and following directions.

Level 5 and 6 Groups

Levels 5 and 6 are introduced to more complex tasks in groups. Some activities suggested are clay and mosaics, cooking and advanced crafts. While one step, demonstrated directions are not necessary, the use of tools and procedures must still be demonstrated at level 5. Several steps can be taught at one time, and patients are capable of selecting projects, and varying colors and designs. Planning is involved and projects may continue for more than one session. The occupational therapist still needs to monitor safety and check understanding of directions, especially with regard to the intangible variables of time and temperature.

Cognitive Behavioral Concepts

Unlike behavior modification which puts the control in the hands of the therapist and external forces, cognitive behavioral therapies seek to modify how a person thinks. Rather than just a stimulus and response continuum, thought processes are inserted between the two. The stimulus involves a situation and an emotion or feeling state; then an analysis of both the situation and the feeling occurs in which various response behaviors are considered and their consequences anticipated. Only after such an analysis does a behavioral response occur. Cognitive therapists seek to discover the thought processes of patients and to help patients use their own cognitive abilities to dispute thinking patterns which lead to problematic behaviors.

Three major contributors to the psychological cognitive behavioral theory are identified by Bruce and Borg (1987) as Albert Bandura, Aaron Beck and Albert Ellis.

Bandura–Social Learning Theory

Bandura's best known contribution to cognitive behavioral theory is his social learning theory (1977, 78). The major areas of focus in Bandura's work are: the role of internal and external reinforcers, mediating environment and person interactions, modeling and observation learning, self-control and self-regulation, and alternative sources of motivation.

Regarding reinforcement, Bandura contends that the person as well as the environment determines behavior. A social learning interaction invloves three factors: person, behavior and environment. External reinforcers are measurable outcomes from the environment, such as getting a grade on a test. The person's interpretation and expectations are considered equally important; these are the internal reinforcers. Examples of external reinforcers are money, material goods, social approval or privileges and penalties. Bandura names two kinds of internal reinforcers: vicarious and self-produced. Vicarious reinforcers are symbolic, such as a person's learned images of success and failure, or reflections of his values and ideals. Self-produced reinforcers come from the persons' sense of competence, efficacy and self-control. In other words, feeling good about oneself is reinforcing.

Hierarchy of Reinforcement

Bandura's heirarchy of reinforcement is helpful in understanding and planning learning experiences for our patient groups. The levels of reinforcers progress from simple to more complex as they parallel the developmental sequence.

1) Initial reinforcers refers to the external ones such as food, attention and approval.
2) Symbolic reinforcers are internal images or messages regarding probable consequences of behavior. An example of this is a child refraining from going outside his yard because he remembers the how angry his mother got the last time he did it.
3) Social contract refers to more complex or role dependent behavior such as performing a job or honoring one's marriage vows.
4) Personal satisfaction is the best and most effective reinforcer in Bandura's opinion, because it is the least dependent upon external circumstances, and therefore the least vulnerable to extinction. When feelings of self-satisfaction or self-worth result from particular behaviors, those behaviors tend to be repeated.

Person-Environment Interactions

The role of cognition in mediating environment and person interactions is another important component in social learning theory. Bandura contends that behavior is an interacting determinant of the outcome or response. For example, a group member's behavior might elicit anger in the other group members. Cognition affects the person in his beliefs about himself and the group. Sam believes he is not an alcoholic, but that others in the group are alcoholics. This belief leads him to reflect an aloof attitude toward other members. When they ask him to participate, he refuses, and he will not respond to the comments of others. The group members interpret his behavior as critical of them - "he thinks he's better than we are." This makes them respond to Sam with anger. Sam hears their angry comments and feels rejected; he logically concludes that the group is not interested in him or able to help him. All of these processes, beliefs and attitudes, interpretations and logical conclusions are cognitive processes that influence the person-environment interaction. In using this concept with Allen's level 5 and 6 patients, group leaders can facilitate an analysis of social interactions that encourages the uncovering of underlying beliefs and attitudes. These patients may be able to use this process to question their own attitudes and change beliefs that are troublesome.

Modeling and Observation Learning

Modeling and observation learning are types of social learning which all persons engage in throughout life. Yet people don't imitate every behavior they see. Cognition plays a major role in the analysis of observed behavior and the selection of which behavior to model. Bandura contends that this selection depends upon anticipated consequences. This means that individuals seek to model behavior which they have observed to have positive consequences. Occupational therapy group leaders can use this process to great advantage. Leaders can model positive responses to others, effective interactions and successful problem-solving, for example. This technique helps patients to increase their own interactional and problem-solving skills. Modeling and imitation are useful even at Allen's lower cognitive levels, beginning at level two where imitation of gross movement improves function. However, the selection process involving anticipation of consequences is not possible until level six.

Self-Control and Self-Regulation

Self-control and self-regulation are desired outcomes of therapy. The basic assumption is that persons are in control of their own behavior and can influence the outcome of their treatment. Cognition influences their motivation, selection of goals and the ability to achieve them. Goals can serve as guides for self-regulation. Persons can measure their own progress in terms of desired goals. Goals are always central in a cognitive behavioral approach to group treatment. The goals of the group are shared with patients and agreed upon at the outset. Activities of the group are directed toward the goal(s) and numbers often evaluate the group in terms of progress toward the goal. Since goals are clearly stated, progress can be easily tested and reported by the therapist. This is partly what makes this approach so useful in acute care settings where gains are expected to be made quickly and progress is evaluated on a daily basis. This concept begins to apply at Allen's cognitive level four, for which goal directed behavior is possible.

Cognition also influences the development of insight or self understanding. Educating patients in how they might analyze their own attitudes, behavior and consequences will enhance their ability to regulate their own behavior. When an anxious patient understands the forces in the environment and the beliefs in himself that contribute to his anxiety, that patient can more easily exercise self-control. He can regulate the situation by reconsidering the reality of his beliefs or removing himself to a less stressful environment. For example, Amy, a college student, studies in her room where her roommate constantly irritates her by playing loud music. Amy believes she can't study with loud music playing. If she changes her attitude, she may learn to enjoy the music or she may be able to view it as a screen for other more distracting noises. If Amy can't do this, she may choose to study in the library.

Beck - Cognitive Therapy

Aaron Beck developed his methods of cognitive behavioral therapy in the 60's and 70's through his work with depressed patients. His approach is founded in empirical investigation: he treats the patient's maladaptive interpretations and conclusions about events as hypotheses to be tested. Beck collaborates with the patient in conducting behavioral experiments, verbal examinations of alternative interpretations, reality testing and problem-solving. From this description it is evident that only patients who are at Allen's highest cognitive levels would be capable of this complex self-analysis.

From his clinical findings, Beck concludes that psychological disturbances frequently stem from habitual errors in thinking. This cognitive model does not assume that the cognitions operate exclusive of biochemistry or behavior symptomatic of psychopathology. Cognition is considered the problem and not the cause. The structure and process of cognitive therapy includes setting the agenda for the session, eliciting feedback, setting goals for therapy, operationally defining problems, testing hypotheses, problem-solving techniques and assigning homework. This structure lends itself very well to occupational therapy groups which can address through activities the cognitive roadblocks to functional performance.

Ellis - Rational Emotive Therapy

Albert Ellis is well known for his work in rational emotive therapy (RET). Although Ellis and Beck developed their techniques over approximately the same time period, each has his own somewhat eclectic basis of which traditional behavior therapy is only a part. Like Beck, Ellis considered thinking to be a legitimate behavior which could be learned and modified using behavior modification techniques. A distinguishing feature of RET is it's systematic exposition of irrational beliefs that result in emotional and behavioral disturbances. Ellis spends most of his energy looking for "unconditional shoulds" and "absolute musts." He contends that patients take "simple preferences" such as desire for love, approval and success and make the mistake of thinking of them as dire needs.

Ellis's view of human nature is somewhat humanistic: he believes people have inborn tendencies toward growth and actualization. He takes for granted, however, that humans are fallible and often make mistakes resulting in "crooked thinking" and "self-defeating" behavior (Ellis, 1973). RET has developed into a kind of structured challenging and disputing of irrational beliefs. It's confrontive methodology, such as the use of exaggeration, absurdity and humor, is not at all humanistic.

RET is a philosophical restructuring process involving a series of steps, all of which require high level thinking.

1) acknowledging our responsibility for creating our own problems;
2) accepting our ability to change our own problems;
3) seeing that emotional problems stem from irrational beliefs;
4) clearly perceiving our beliefs;
5) rigorously disputing beliefs;
6) working hard to change beliefs resulting in disturbed emotion and behavior;
7) practicing RET methods over our lifetime.

RET is very much a skill development process to be used over one's lifetime (Ellis & Harper, 1975). The therapist teaches the client how to apply a scientific approach to thinking. The therapist acts as an educator-facilitator in collaborating with the client to achieve specific goals. In occupational therapy groups, when we use a psychoeducational approach, our role as educator-facilitator is similar to that outlined by Ellis and Beck. Our goal is to teach skills that can be generalized by patients after they leave therapy groups. Groups that focus on stress management, time management, leisure planning and health education are examples of OT groups using a cognitive behavioral approach. Discussion of the problems patients have in the performance leads to exposure of faulty thinking. In our higher functioning patient groups, OT's can help the patients change their attitudes toward disability or ability as it effects performance. We can teach our group members to challenge each other and to encourage their use of rational thinking to solve problems.

Function and Dysfunction

A well-functioning individual has the ability to think logically and to form accurate perceptions of the self and the environment. He/she can use deductive reasoning to cope with problems and can logically regulate his/her own thoughts and behavior. Allen has been concerned with competence, which legally means the ability to handle one's own affairs. There is no cut-off cognitive level for defining competence. Determination of competence or incompetence are generally based on the ability to make sound judgments and reasonable decisions about those activities that the individual intends to do.

Dysfunction is characterized by limitations in conscious awareness, faulty thinking, inaccurate self-perception and the inability to handle one's affairs competently. Failure to adapt to the environment and to function independently in society in this frame of reference is seen as a product of cognitive disability. Therefore it is cognitive impairments in attention, sensory awareness, perception, thought processes, problem solving and learning new coping strategies that are the cause of problems in doing functional activities. These cognitive functions, therefore, should be the focus of treatment in occupational therapy.

Change and Motivation

In both the cognitive disabilities and the cognitive behavioral approach, people change by changing the way they think. For higher cognitive levels, Allen's levels 5 and 6, becoming aware of beliefs and attitudes that result in problem emotions and behaviors is the first step. Challenging these "faulty thoughts" can convince patients to change them, and this will lead to a change in behavior. The occupational therapist can use this educational approach to teach patients to apply logic to produce adaptive change, when their patients' disability does not affect cognition, such as patients with arthritis or hand injury, or those suffering from substance abuse.

When cognitive processes are damaged by trauma or disease, Allen suggests that we can still produce changes in adaptive functioning by manipulating the environment. In doing a task, there are several factors to be manipulated. The task environment includes materials, lighting, seating, facilities available, and assistance available. The task demand is the instructions and the difficulty of the processes necessary to complete the task. Allen suggests that both the task environment and the task demand can be altered in ways that allow the patient to perform more independently within his cognitive level. For example, a level 4 patient's adaptive functioning can reach its maximum by providing a task that is within his or her ability, setting out all the necessary materials within his or her visual field, and demonstrating the instructions one step at a time (with a completed sample for him to copy). This patient can perform most self-care tasks at home with appropriate assistance and a suitable and safe environment.

It is assumed that people have a natural drive toward competence and mastery, and to achieve a better position in life. People wish to be self-directed and to have an effect on others and on the environment. To achieve these goals, most people are willing to learn and try new coping strategies for problem-solving and for self-improvement/regulation. A difficulty with this approach may be to find effective reinforcements for those patients that do not seem to be motivated, or are unaware of a social pressure to improve their status.

Group Treatment

Two somewhat divergent approaches have been described in the theoretical section of this chapter. Both share the basic assumptions about the nature of man, disability and the role of assessment and treatment. By now it should be clear that the kind of therapies described by Beck, Bandura and Ellis have limitations in application, as does Allen's approach. The kind of logical, scientific thinking required to participate in cognitive behavioral therapy is fairly high-level, and is quite beyond the scope of the average schizophrenic or dementia patient. Claudia Allen's more concrete activities approach at the lower and middle cognitive levels seems quite effective for these patients. But the project-centered approach may fail to challenge the level 5 and 6 patient, who may not have any limitations in performance of visual/spacial tasks. Accordingly, occupational therapists, in using a cognitive behavioral approach, should use the psychoeducational model for higher functioning patients, while reserving Allen's guidelines for lower functioning patients.

Larger numbers of patients can be treated at once in this frame of reference. Earhart (Allen 1985) suggests up to 20 at a time, with two therapists supervising. The group is usually highly structured, with concentrated work toward a specific goal as the focus. It is most often suggested in the literature that groups be formed homogeneously, that is, patients with similar problems and goals or patients functioning at the same cognitive level are grouped together. Efficiency in goal attainment is all-important, and the OT structures the group and the environment with this in mind.

Role of the Leader

The occupational therapist's role is more directive in this frame of reference than it is in most others. In a hospital setting the focus is often on evaluation. The therapist typically chooses the activity or task, or limits choices. The OT becomes the expert in activity analysis, controlling the environment and teaching the skills that the task demands. The therapist's role is active in giving assistance or promoting patients to a higher cognitive level.

The role softens in rehabilitation and custodial care situations; setting treatment goals with patients becomes a collaborative process between therapist, patient and other care givers. In groups of patients and care givers, mutual problem solving to adapt intended activities for the health and safety of the individual with a residual disability is the focus of care. Bruce and Borg (1987) point out that the therapist's role is that of an "educator-facilitator" in the psychoeducational groups. For example, in a health education group for levels 5 and 6, the occupational therapist may survey the needs of the group and then present a series of short lectures based on the group need to learn about health maintenance.

Goals of the Group

For the higher level patients who might seek rational emotive therapy skills (Ellis) or cognitive therapy (Beck), the goal is insight. Only when a patient understands the impact of his negative self statements and harsh self-judgments is he/she able or willing to change them. It is assumed that a change in thinking will produce a change in behavior. Therefore goals will generally address the thought processes rather than the affective or overt behavioral components.

Allen's goals for patients have to do with function and adaptation. Specific goals might be set to encourage a patient to progress to a higher level, or to provide the ideal environmental support and assistance so that a patient can maximize function within a given cognitive level. Allen has designed several excellent evaluation tools, and specified many behaviors that indicate progress toward higher cognitive levels.

One contribution of the cognitive behavioral frame of reference is the concept of behavioral goals. The goals for our occupational therapy groups should be written in specific, measurable terms. Often these goals are set by the patients and therapist together, and progress toward the goals is openly discussed with the group. In cognitive behavioral groups, an evaluation of the group should be set up to see if goals are met. The following exercises are designed to help students learn how to write behavioral goals.

Exercise 1
Writing Long Term Goals

Directions: Begin by writing your lifetime goals for yourself. Write at least one goal from each of the following categories:

1. professional

2. educational

3. monetary

4. family

5. health

6. social

7. spiritual

8. emotional

9. recreational

10. creative

Long-term goals are not always measurable. Sometimes when we set lifetime goals, such as "be successful at my job", it is not clear what it is that success really means. Even when these goals are measurable, such as "become a millionaire by age 40," how these goals will be accomplished remains unplanned. Until these goals are broken down into smaller, do-able steps, they will remain only dreams. Short-term, measurable goals are the actions and behaviors that help us and our patients make dreams a reality. A measurable goal is one that describes behavior that can be observed. For example, your goal might be to improve self-esteem. How can you tell when self-esteem has improved? What behaviors would you look for? What actions could you take? Some possibilities might be standing taller, taking more care in dressing and hygiene to look your best, and verbalizing several positive aspects of yourself.

Exercise 2
Recognizing Measurable Goals

Directions: From the list below, check off the goals that you think are measurable.

1. encourage decision making

2. list one strength and one weakness

3. develop a better self-concept

4. discuss feelings about parents

5. relate better to authority figures

6. manage time better

7. conserve energy in cooking a meal

8. handle frustration

9. demonstrate pride in personal accomplishment

10. plan a weekend activity and carry it out

11. define assertive behavior

12. complete a task within time limit

13. relieve stress

14. eat a well-balanced diet

15. plan time to study for a test

16. take responsibility for behavior

17. attend school regularly

18. stay on a diet 80% of the time

19. understand yourself better

20. strengthen feminine/masculine identity

The measurable goals in Exercise 2 are 2, 4, 9, 10, 12, 14, 15, 17, and 18. One key to writing a measurable goal is the language used. Words like learn, understand, encourage, improve, handle and manage are vague because they don't specify how these things can be accomplished. Measurable goals are usually specific, and they incorporate behaviors that can be observed. Words like define, list, discuss and complete refer to either words or actions which can be readily observed, heard or read. In the cognitive behavioral frame of reference, thoughts are also considered to be behavior. However, thoughts must be verbalized in order to be measurable.

Exercise 3
Making Our Lifetime Goals Measurable

Directions: In Exercise 1, we wrote down some lifetime goals. First, go back to that list and check off which of those goals are measurable. Next, choose three goals from your list which are *not* measurable and write them down below. For each one, list several measurable short-term goals or steps to be completed.

Lifetime goal #1 _____

    a. _____

    b. _____

    c. _____

    d. _____

    e. _____

Lifetime goal #2 _____

    a. _____

    b. _____

    c. _____

    d. _____

    e. _____

Lifetime goal #3 _____

    a. _____

    b. _____

    c. _____

    d. _____

    e. _____

Examples of Activities

Occupational therapists may borrow and adapt many specific techniques from cognitive behaviorism to enhance our activity groups. Some of these techniques should be recognized as very powerful and therefore dangerous to use without specific training. Some of the techniques OTs should avoid unless specifically trained are flooding, paradoxical intention and systematic desensitization. These techniques involve vivid imaging of much-feared and disturbing situations, and the management of patients who have been so aroused requires more advanced therapeutic skills.

However, in moderation, imaging and visualization may be incorporated into a structured activity or may be expanded into drawing, sculpture or dramatic role play. The use of images or visualization is a technique many occupational therapists have found helpful. For example, the guided fantasy can enhance relaxation and foster creativity and self-awareness. Once goals are set, visualizing images of their successful achievement is often motivating. Drawing images of various kinds is one way to structure our groups to work on specific goals.

The concepts of group problem-solving, keeping journals and giving homework are also useful ideas in occupational therapy groups. Behavior rehearsal may be useful in the learning and practice of social skills. Some other techniques are: contracts with oneself or with the group to change certain thoughts and behavior, self-reward or self-punishment, writing beliefs in words and then deciding if the statements are true or false, positive or negative labeling of thoughts, feelings and behavior. The reader is referred to McMullin (1986) *Handbook of Cognitive Therapy Techniques* for more ideas.

Any activity which can help patients learn coping skills is fair game. Structured activities that address values clarification, assertiveness training, stress management, relaxation, and time management are some popular examples. Self-care skills, work skills, leisure activities and social skills can also be learned effectively using a cognitive behavioral approach. Here are some examples of cognitive behavioral groups.

Setting Priorities

This activity has been used as the first session of a time management workshop for substance abuse patients. It serves as an ice breaker for patients who do not know each other well, and also helps the therapist to formulate goals for the group.

Materials: Values Survey Worksheets, pencils

Directions: Often the things we spend our time doing are not the things we want most to do. Setting priorities means deciding what is important to us, and doing that first. As a first step in helping to plan our time better, we will look at what we value.

1. (Pass out Values Survey Worksheets) Take the next ten minutes to think about the values listed, and number them according to their order of importance to you. Put number 1 next to the most important item, number 2 for the next level of importance, and so forth, up to number 8 for the least important. Do not use the same number more than once.
2. Ask each member to share their top three values and discuss in what way these values are a part of his/her life right now.
3. Write your top three values on the lower section of the Values Survey Worksheet, and below each write one specific goal that reflects that value. For example, if "freedom to do what I want" is one of your values, your goal might be to move out of your parents' house and get your own apartment. You have five minutes for this part.
4. Looking at your goals, choose one to work on this weekend. At the bottom of the worksheet, write down one activity that you can plan this weekend to help you accomplish the goal.

Values Survey Worksheet

Directions: Eight commonly held values are listed here. Think about your own life in relation to these values. Then give each a number, beginning with number 1 for the most important to you, number 2 for the second most important and so forth, up to number 8 for the least important. Do not use any number more than once.

_____ A good love relationship

_____ Financial security

_____ A satisfying religious faith

_____ Freedom to do what I want

_____ Meaningful family life

_____ Success at my chosen career

_____ Excitement and adventure

_____ Making lots of money

First most important value _____

Goal: _____

_____

Second most important value_____

Goal: _____

_____

Third most important value_____

Goal: _____

_____

Planned activity to work on goal _____

_____

_____

Telling Others About Your Illness

This activity has been part of a patient group on coping with illness. The group is given short lectures each week on a different aspect of coping with illness, followed by participation in a related activity.

Materials: two chairs placed in center of the group

Directions: Each patient will take a turn sitting in the chair in the center. First, the patient will tell the group what his/her illness is, and why it is difficult to talk to others about it. Then the patient will choose another member to play the part of a relative or friend. The therapist is the "director" and directs as follows:

Friend or relative: Ask how the patient is and ask follow-up questions.

Patient: Answer him/her as if it were a real conversation.

Patient: Now change places with your friend and respond for him/her. Now change places again and be yourself again. Try to tell your friend how you "feel" about being ill. Try to keep each conversation going for about five minutes. Members should volunteer for this and no one should be forced.

After each discussion, the group is asked to respond and to discuss the role play. Were the players being "genuine"? Were feelings being expressed freely? What are other ways to make the discussion helpful?

Relaxation Fantasy Activity

This activity has been a part of a stress management group in which members use the techniques of visualization and guided fantasy to control their state of tension.

Materials: Carpeted open space, patients wearing sweatsuits and sneakers or other comfortable clothing, pillows for each person.

Directions: Members sit in a circle on the floor, pillows in their laps. They should be far enough apart that all can lie down and reach out their arms without touching one another.
1. Introduction: Relaxation is as much in your mind as in your body. Therefore, if you want to be relaxed, and free your body from stress, your mind must take the lead. It is very difficult to feel relaxed when your mind is preoccupied with worry. As you do this exercise, try to concentrate on the visual images that come into your head. Instructions will be given for you to move your physical position as well as parts of your body. Try to do these with your eyes closed, so you will not lose the mental images created.
2. You are about to take a 30 minute relaxation break from your busy, stressful or boring day. Maybe you have a lot of work to do, or a difficult situation to face. Put that out of your mind for the next 30 minutes. Afterward, when you are relaxed, you'll have more energy to cope with life's hassles.
3. Begin by reaching both arms up over your head in a big stretch. Open your mouth wide and yawn. Now place the pillow behind your hips and lean back on your elbows. Close your eyes and imagine a door far across the room in front of you.

Without moving your position, imagine yourself walking toward the door. Move your feet, your ankles, your knees and your hips as if you were walking. When the right leg is tense, allow the left one to relax. Now point your toes each time you take a "step." Slow down your steps and inhale as you tense your right leg, then exhale as you tense your left leg. As you approach the door, your steps become slower and slower (2 minutes). When you reach the door, stand in front of it and continue breathing slowly.

4. Push yourself up with your arms to a sitting position. With your eyes still closed, lean forward and peek through a small hole in the door. You see a welcome view. It is a lovely, sunny patio with a sparkling in-ground pool. It is surrounded by clean, comfortable lounge chairs. Keep your hands behind you on the floor as you lean forward to get a better view. Stretch your back and push yourself forward with your arms until you feel the stretch behind your thighs. Keep breathing slowly.

5. With eyes still closed, bend your knees up to your chest. With one hand gripping each knee, imagine that your knees are the handles of the door. Pull gently on the "handles", straightening your back as you pull. Then let go as the door opens wide. As you pass through the door, you leave behind all the worries of the day. On the other side of the door there are no worries, no stress, so let them all go.

6. Without opening your eyes, straighten your legs and move the pillow under your head as you lie down on one of the comfortable lounge chairs. The sun feels good as it warms you. Imagine you are wearing a bathing suit under your sweatshirt. While still lying down, pretend to take the sweatshirt off. First, put hands near hips and push down on elbows to raise hips slightly off the floor. Then raise hands up to chest level, elbows still on the floor. Push head back into the pillow as you raise shoulders slightly off the floor. Pause here and breathe. Now raise your head off the pillow as you pretend to lift the sweatshirt off over your head and let it drop to the ground behind your pillow. This done, slowly return arms to your sides while breathing out slowly. Just lay there breathing slowly, enjoying the warm sun (2 minutes).

7. Check your body to be sure it's relaxed. Wiggle your fingers and your toes. Roll your head to the right, then roll your head to the left. If there's tension anywhere, shake it out. Put your hand behind your neck and massage your neck muscles. Keep breathing slowly. It feels so relaxing to lie here in the warm sun (2 minutes).

8. The sun is getting hot now. Maybe it's time to go for a swim. Raise yourself up to a sitting position again and bring your knees up to your chest. Now imagine you're sitting on the edge of the pool. Dangle your legs into the pleasantly cool water. Turn around to the left and look behind you; turn around to the right and look behind you. The signs say Good Swimming Today, so turn over slowly onto your stomach as you lower yourself into the water.

9. As you float on your stomach, your pillow has become a life preserver. Hold onto the pillow as you kick your legs slowly, floating around the pool. Your feet need not even leave the floor. It takes almost no effort at all to move you through the water. Your body doesn't feel heavy. Now inhale as you kick your right leg, exhale as you kick your left leg. As you reach the edge of the pool, push away again, continuing to hold onto the life preserver with one hand, then the other.

10. Now lift up on your elbows and push the pillow down under your ribcage, so it supports your chest as you lean on your elbows. Continue to breathe slowly. Shrug your shoulders up toward your ears, then release. Shrug away your last bit of tension. Now you are relaxed, refreshed and energetic. Now you are capable of

resuming your day without feeling tension and stress. Miraculously, you are out of the pool, dry and dressed again, standing in front of the door. Now you feel prepared to go back through that door and take on the world. When you are ready, open your eyes.

Falling Leaves

This is a basic craft group for Allen's cognitive level 4 patients. It is a group project following the guidelines of task analysis presented by Claudia Allen (1985).

Materials: The table is set up by the therapist for 6-10 patients. Half of the patients have a sheet of colored paper, a pencil, a pair of paper scissors and a cardboard pattern of a leaf. Leaf shapes used are maple, elm, oak, ash, tulip, and birch. Real leaves can be traced to produce these patterns. However, this is done by the therapist. The other half of the patients have a piece of white poster board with a tree trunk and branches traced in black magic marker and the name of the tree outlined in black. Chunky capital letters are best, saying OAK, MAPLE, etc. with the centers to be colored in. Patients with the tree trunks also have two wide tip markers, brown or gray and another color, and a small bottle of glue.

Directions: Therapist should demonstrate the processes.

1. Leaves. Place the leaf pattern on the colored paper and trace around it with the pencil. Fit as many as you can on the paper without overlapping any lines. When finished cut out each leaf along the lines you have traced.
2. Tree trunks. Color in the tree trunk with the appropriate color. Then color in the letters with another color. When finished, glue the appropriate leaves on the tree branches. Patients may work in pairs, so that maple leaves are glued to the maple tree trunk, etc. Colors of the leaves should be appropriate for autumn. For variation, two autumn shades may be used for each leaf to create a more interesting pattern.

Discussion will center around the autumn season, what happens in the fall, and what kinds of tasks must be done to prepare for the autumn/winter season. The tree posters make a good decoration for the ward.

Building Our Community

This activity is part of a psychoeducational group focusing on independent living skills with chronic schizophrenic patients. The goal of this session is to help the group become aware of community resources.

Materials: One square of 1/4" plywood, approximately 30" x 30", a variety of small blocks of scrap wood with rough edges and splinters sanded off, jars of poster paint in several colors, brushes, and wood glue. This project may take two sessions to complete.

Directions:

1. The group begins by discussing the communities they live in and what services and resources are available there. The occupational therapist helps the group develop a list of services they need to have available in their community. A typical list includes

a hospital, grocery store, department store, drug store, police department, fire department, school, movie theater, etc. Why they need each one and how they would use them is discussed.

Figure 5-1. Our Community.

2. Next, the group members build from the blocks a community they would like to live in. Each member chooses one or more community resources to build, and constructs a school, a movie theater, etc. by gluing blocks together. The "buildings" are then painted and colored signs are painted on to label them. Buildings are then placed and glued onto the plywood square, something like an architect's model city. Streets, parking lots, parks, or bodies of water may be painted directly on the plywood if desired. (My thanks to D.M. Hancock, OT student at Quinnipiac, for this creative idea.)

Group Leadership

The seven step group format is not changed in structure. If anything, in this frame of reference, groups become even more structured. Some of the discussion portions may be eliminated for patients at Allen's level 4 and below. The beginning of the group places an emphasis on defining specific problems and collaborative goal setting. The therapist may do this individually before the group begins.

Introduction

This kind of group will dispense with the warm-up and get right down to business. A more complete explanation of the goals and purpose will substitute. Expectations are spelled out in behavioral terms, and the group is told how their progress will be evaluated. The time frame of the group should coincide with the members' level of cognitive functioning. Lower levels (Allen's level 3, for example), may last only 30 minutes, while higher levels go up to 90 minutes.

Activity

Cognitive behavioral groups focus on learning coping skills and improving task performance. There is usually didactic instruction given in the form of short lectures or demonstrations of the steps in doing a task. The activities are learning experiences and opportunities for practice. In a leisure skills group, for example, members learn to do a series of specific activities: how to knit, how to cook, how to catch a fish, how to play card games. In a stress management group, the occupational therapist gives mini-lessons in cardiovascular fitness, high nutrition diets and progressive relaxation in conjunction with activities. The experience may take longer, up to two-thirds of the session, leaving the rest for discussion/demonstration.

Sharing

This part is minimized, since members essentially work on their own projects and problems. However, feedback from others is an important social reinforcement to learning, and should be offered to all members. Feedback comes mostly from the therapist in the lower level groups, and from fellow members in higher level groups.

Processing

Discussion of the underlying dynamics of the group is also not an area of focus. Most of the interaction should be between the leader and each member, just as a teacher interacts with a class. However, when the feelings or the implicit forces of the group begin to interfere with group learning, then the therapist must temporarily make group process the focus.

Generalizing

Inductive reasoning is encouraged in the members to come up with general principles to be learned from the experience. Inductive reasoning involves collecting evidence from many specific examples to build a general principle or theory. Members can do this best when they have heard several responses to the experience from other members. In a well-planned group, the general principles suggested by the members will coincide with group goals. If this does not happen spontaneously, the therapist should help the group to make the connections. Generalizing is not possible in groups of patients at Allen's level 4 and below.

Application

There is more emphasis here than in any other part of the discussion. An effective group will include a carry-over of behavior change from the clinic to the community environment. Members should know before they leave the group exactly how they will apply their new knowledge or skill. Members may share ideas on how to do this. The activities done by the group are usually planned to address specific problems, so the application is generally built into the group experience at the outset. Homework may be given by the therapist to support the application of what is learned.

Summary

The main purpose of the summary is to reinforce learning. It is best done by the therapist in most cases. Reminders about homework and announcements about what is planned next are also appropriate.

Bibliography

Allen C. *Occupational therapy for psychiatric diseases.* Boston/Toronto: Little, Brown & Co., 1985.

Allen C. and Allen R. Cognitive disabilities: Measuring the social consequences of mental disorders. *J. Clinical Psychiatry,* 1987, 48,5,185-190.

Allen C. and Earhart K. *OT Treatment Goals for the Physically and Cognitively Disabled.* Rockville, MD: AOTA, 1992.

Allen C. and Earhart K. *Expanded Activities Analysis.* Pasadena, CA: authors, 1988.

Bandura A. *Social Learning Theory.* Englewood Cliffs, NJ: Prentice-Hall, 1977.

Beck A. *Cognitive Therapy and Emotional Disorders.* NY: Intl. Univ. Press, 1976.

Bruce M. and Borg B. *Frames of Reference in Psychosocial Occupational Therapy.* Thorofare, NJ: SLACK Inc., 1987.

Corey G. *Theory and Practice of Counseling and Psychotherapy* (4th ed.). Monterrey, CA: Brooks/Cole, 1991.

Dryden W. and Golden W. *Cognitive-Behavioral Approaches to Psychotherapy.* London: Harper & Row, 1986.

Ellis A. *Humanistic Psychology: The Rational Emotive Approach.* NY: McGraw-Hill, 1973.

Ellis A. and Harper R. *A New Guide to Rational Living.* No. Hollywood, CA: Wilshire Book Company, 1975.

McMullin R.E. *Handbook of Cognitive Behavioral Techniques,* NY: Norton, 1986.

Mosey A. *Psychosocial Components of Occupational Therapy,* NY: Raven, 1986.

Chapter

6

A Developmental Approach

This chapter focuses on developmental theory as it applies to adults. Although some of the theorists deal primarily with children, it is assumed that disease and injury interfere with development in ways that affect them as adults. The guiding principle of all developmental theories is that there is a developmental sequence from birth to maturity and throughout life to death. This sequence is determined by both biological and environmental forces. This development occurs in stages, which are **specific, progressive** and **hierarchical**. Development is divided into stages for the benefit of our understanding. In reality, the transition from one stage to the next is gradual. Each stage, however, is subdivided into specific skills, issues or conflicts and each has characteristics that distinguish it from other stages.

Progressive stages refer to the idea that each stage increases in complexity and represents, in some way, progress toward maturity. It is assumed that maturity is the highest stage, and therefore the goal. Maturity is seen in both an individual and a social context. In other words, the goal of maturity may be the survival and success of the individual, but maturity also involves cooperation with others and the survival and flourishing of humanity. Hierarchical stages mean that each stage builds on the next. It reinforces the idea that there are foundation skills upon which higher level skills are built. According to developmental theory, skills which are deficient must be learned in the same sequence in which they normally develop. This idea seems common to all the theorists reviewed here.

Basic Assumptions

There are many different theories of human development, some ending with adolescence (Freud), and others continuing right through old age (Erikson, Jung). Those discussed here are chosen because they help clarify our thinking about occupational therapy groups. Included are Jung, Erikson, Levinson, Kohlberg and Wilcox and Gilligan. Some of the theories of physiological and cognitive development, such as Ayres and Piaget, have been eliminated here and are covered instead in the next chapter on the neurodevelopmental frame of reference.

Jung

Jung, who wrote in the 1940s and '50s, might be considered the father of adult development theory. He differed from Freud in extending the developmental process throughout life, and acknowledging the contribution of external factors to growth and adaptation. Jung divided life into four basic stages: childhood, youth, mid-life and old age. In Jung's view, childhood is spent in blissful ignorance. Although influenced by many inherited predispositions, children develop with no doubts, unaware of their own growth processes. Youth is marked by the onset of consciousness, of doubts, problems, contradictions and responsibilities. Jung described the second half of life as beginning between ages 35 and 40, when the essential character of life changes and energy becomes rechanneled. Before age 40, the individual has put his energy into external events such as establishing occupation, community position, marriage and family. After age 40, Jung believes the individual turns inward, focusing more on the spiritual (Schultz 1976).

Middle age is described by Jung as the "afternoon of life." Polarities are opposite tendencies of the self present in an individual, such as introversion vs. extroversion, rationality vs. intuitiveness, aggressiveness vs. sensitivity and action vs. contemplation. At mid-life, Jung contends that whatever sides of the self were expressed in the person's youth, the opposite sides will prevail in mid-life. It was Jung who identified individuation as the true goal of life, a concept much in question in the 1980s. Individuation is a kind of enhancement of identity which involves further definition of the self. Individuation continues through each of the stages in greater depths and in different ways. The end result of individuation was thought to be integration, a uniting of all parts of the self into a qualified whole.

Old age is the final stage. As a person ages he faces physical decline, removes himself from positions of authority and responsibility and faces the inevitability of his own death. Jung assumed a belief in the presence of an afterlife, and began the idea that all individuals ultimately contribute to a "collective unconscious," and so live on through others. (Table 6-1.)

Erikson

Erikson also built on Freud's psychosexual stages, and extended his theory to include adolescence and adulthood. His ideas are compatible with Jung's, but more social in nature and based on the central issues of each stage as conflicts to be resolved. The stages which most impact our adult patient groups are: identity vs. role confusion—ages 13 to 21, intimacy vs. isolation—ages 19 to 35, generativity vs. stagnation—ages 35 to 50 and integrity vs. despair—ages 50 to death. Erikson's stages are well-known and referred to

Table 6-1.
Jung's Stages of Development (Spiritual)

Age	Stage
Birth to Puberty (Childhood)	Blissful ignorance, inherited predispositions
Puberty to Age 35 (Youth)	Conscious and doubting, taking on responsiblity
Age 35 to old age (Midlife)	Change in direction to express latent parts of self individuation and integration
Infirmity and Death (Old Age)	Infirmity, acceptance of death, afterlife and collective unconscious

often in occupational therapy literature. The conflict areas can guide our choice of activities in occupational therapy and can serve as a basis for setting goals at the various age levels. For example, trust issues can be worked on through movement activities, such as "falling" and "being caught," or through verbal activities, such as giving and receiving emotional support. (Table 6-2.)

Table 6-2.
Erikson's Eight Stages of Development (Psychosocial)

Age	Stage
Birth - Infancy	Trust vs. Mistrust
2-4 Toddlerhood	Autonomy vs. Shame and Doubt
5-7 Early childhood	Initiative vs. Guilt
8-12 Middle child	Industry vs. Inferiority
13-22 Adolescence	Identity vs. Role Diffusion
23-35 Young Adult	Intimacy vs. Isolation
35-50 Adulthood	Generativity vs. Stagnation
50-Death	Integrity vs. Despair

Levinson

Levinson (1978) has published the most extensive (although admittedly controversial) research study to date on the developmental stages of adulthood. He based his findings on a longevity study of 40 men. Levinson presents adulthood as periods of stability alternating with periods of transition. The three life transitions he identifies are: early adult—ages 17 to 22, mid-life—ages 40 to 45 and late adult—age 60 to 65 transitions. These periods of conflict are interspersed with periods of relative stability in which the individual lives within an established life structure and stays more or less on course (see Table 6-3).

Levinson contends that each transition period occurs during specific age ranges and each transition has its own developmental tasks. Like Erikson, he saw each transition as requiring the resolution of conflicts before the person can move on to the next stage.

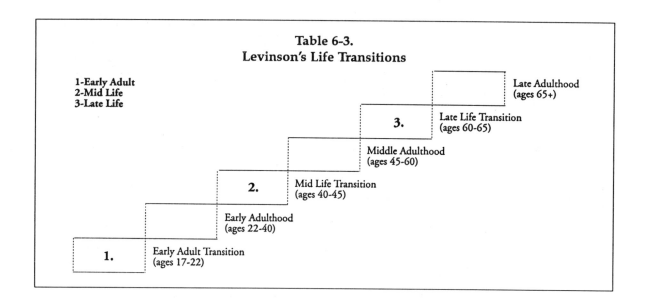

Table 6-3.
Levinson's Life Transitions

1-Early Adult
2-Mid Life
3-Late Life

Late Adulthood
(ages 65+)

3. Late Life Transition
(ages 60-65)

Middle Adulthood
(ages 45-60)

2. Mid Life Transition
(ages 40-45)

Early Adulthood
(ages 22-40)

1. Early Adult Transition
(ages 17-22)

Primarily the tasks of each transition period are to re-evaluate the existing life structure, explore the possibilities of change and make choices that will restructure life in the next era. **Era's** are in between stages of stability described as young, middle and late adulthood. In the Levinson study of 40 men, work was considered to be a "base for life in society" giving the man his life structure in a cultural, class and social sense as well as occupational (Levinson 1978, 9). Since the thrust of the study was to examine the mid-life transition, subjects selected were age 35, from four different occupational groups and were followed to age 45. Biographical information collected from these subjects forms the basis of the young adult transition. The late adult transition is only briefly covered by Levinson and is considered to parallel the preceding transition.

Levinson's theory has been selected for focus because it presents a good structure around which to understand life problems of patients and to plan occupational therapy groups.

The Early Adult Transition

The essence of this transition is the separation from the family of origin in order to establish a new home base. The separation is both geographical and emotional, and generally creates a sense of loss. Yet the excitement involved in establishing oneself in the adult world provides a sense of satisfaction. Exploration in the early adult transition quickly pushes toward commitment as the young man is required to take on adult responsibilities. Balancing exploration with the need for structure is an ongoing struggle. The major tasks of the early adult transition are: forming the dream, finding a mentor, forming an occupation and starting a marriage and family.

Forming the Dream

The first task which plays a powerful role in early adulthood is called forming a dream. Levinson states that the dream emerges during the early adult transition where the boy/man imagines himself settled in the adult world. This may be connected with concrete reality, or far removed from his actual world. The ability to play make believe in early childhood is the forerunner of this imagining in early adulthood. The dream is a vehicle for exploring his image, and "provides a source of hope, self-esteem and personal integrity" (Levinson 1978, 93). The young adult's task includes forming relationships with others who can facilitate his work on the dream and find ways of living it out in his life. If the dream is unconnected with choices made in this stage, it will resurface during the mid-life transition and demand a place for self-expression then.

The Mentor Relationship

According to Levinson, the mentor relationship is very complex and extremely significant for a man during early adulthood. The mentor is a transitional figure in a person's life, serving as a teacher, sponsor, guide and adviser. The most important function of the mentor is "to support and facilitate the realization of the dream" (1978, 98). Offering expertise and counseling to a young man, yet not being parental, the mentor is usually older than his protege by a half-generation. All men in the study had male mentors although Levinson's own mentor was a female, and it is expected that as more women enter currently male-dominated fields, they too will serve as mentors to both men and women.

In a study made by Margaret Hennig of 25 high-level women executives, it was shown that all had found male mentors early in their careers (Sheehy 1976). Interestingly, these successful women chose careers rather than marriage in their 20s, yet realized around age 35 that something was missing and began to explore their feminine sides. Levinson reports a similar happenstance for men who become less involved with their mentors by age 40, and face the task of reintegrating the feminine side of their personality.

Choosing an Occupation

The process of choosing an occupation extends throughout the entire life cycle, beginning in childhood with make-believe games like "doctor," or "teacher." As Levinson remarks about other important life choices, "the great paradox of human development is that we are required to make crucial choices before we have the knowledge, judgment and self-understanding to choose wisely" (1978, 162). Transforming one's early interests into an occupational choice during young adulthood is a complex psychosocial process, and a pattern usually emerges with some definition by the early thirties. An occupation often serves as an index of an individual's worth in society, both economically and socially, and defines his role in the community. For many of the men in Levinson's study, establishing an occupational identity is often tied up with parental expectations, and the nurturing given to the dream concept with or without the presence of a mentor. There are enormous differences between individuals regarding the meaning of success and failure, and concepts around these values change as growth occurs throughout their life span.

This stage has important implications for occupational therapy. Because illness almost always interrupts the work role of the patient, values around self and work need to be reconsidered. Group activities dealing with values around the work role, and the exploration of alternate roles in the home and community are appropriate for a wide variety of patient populations.

Marriage and Family

The developmental task of forming a marriage and family also involves making premature choices. It is unusual to have integrated the many components of a stable adult relationship in the early adulthood stage. Sexuality, dependency, emotional intimacy, friendship and the capability for commitment are but a few of the issues that extend beyond this phase. Actually, the ability to relate to the feminine or masculine aspects of self is a lifetime task, one of the many polarities that both Levinson and Jung give importance to in adult development. Undertaking the obligation to marry and have children does not necessarily mean one is prepared for the responsibilities and commitments. Often this step is intricately bound up with the other tasks of early adulthood, such as separating from parents and finding support for the dream pursuit. Levinson describes a "special woman" (1978, 109) who facilitates a man's entry into the adult world by providing boundaries within which his aspirations can be realized, and giving nourishment to his occupational journey. If the marital choice is made in such a way as to be antithetical to the dream, the relationship may suffer conflicts at a later date. Obviously, the relationship will be modified over time to accommodate the dreams of both the man and woman, and there are endless possibilities for creating a family pattern that is suitable for both. The importance of fatherhood and motherhood may not emerge until the individual has outgrown his occupational mentor and is prepared to provide those types of functions himself to his younger associates and to his own offspring.

The Mid-life Transition

This period is said to provide the bridge from early to middle adulthood. It brings a man to question, search and re-examine his life and his values. For the great majority of men in the Levinson study (80% of subjects), this great struggle within the self and the external world may reach crisis proportions. Often several years are needed to go through the process and come to some resolution. A culminating event often signifies success or failure in the man's fantasy, and this self-judgment may be all encompassing. If he fails to get a promotion, he may regard himself as a failure in other aspects of his life as well. This transition period begins when a man realizes that he cannot go on as before, that he cannot "become his own man" under his existing life structure, and that changes will be necessary in order to advance sufficiently in any chosen direction. Three main tasks are defined by Levinson for this stage of development: 1) to terminate the era of early adulthood (reappraising the past), 2) to take the first steps toward middle adulthood (modifying life structure) and 3) to deal with the polarities that are the sources of deep division in his life (individuation). Each of these broadly defined tasks has many specific aspects to consider.

Reappraising the Past

Recognition of his own mortality gives a man a renewed sense of urgency about the use of his remaining time. He examines his accomplishments in relation to earlier hopes, values and expectations, asking "have I accomplished all that I set out to do?" Because of the nature of a dream, which is essentially fantasy, many ideas, assumptions and beliefs associated with the dream do not withstand the comparison with actual experience. Levinson defines "de-illusionment" as "a recognition that long-held assumptions and beliefs about self and the world are not true" (1978, 192). The process of de-illusionment is accompanied by emotions of disappointment, joy, relief, bitterness, grief, wonder, freedom and pain. At this stage a man may ask: "What have I done with my life? Is what I'm doing now what I want to be doing in the future? Have I reached success at my job? Am I fulfilled by my marital relationship? What are my present values and priorities? Am I spending my time on the things I really value? Is what I have done really meaningful? How have I been fooling myself? (and/or) What is my true worth in my eyes and society's?" Occupational therapy groups can focus on some of these issues to help patients who are facing a mid-life transition to answer some of these questions.

Modifying the Life Structure

Having taken stock of the past, man now begins to plan for the next phase. Exploration of new patterns for living occurs. Some changes are externally motivated. The realities of growing families, aging parents, changes in spouse and the marriage require certain changes in role and point of view. Experience of world politics, economy, cultural and social values also influence the planning of man's new life structure.

But whether or not visible change occurs, one's outlook, values and expectations of life are essentially different as a result of the developmental tasks of the mid-life transition. Questions to be asked are: "What do I want to change in my life? What are my options for change in occupation, marriage and family roles, roles in the community? What are the external changes in my life that put pressure on me to change? What pressures do I feel from society, friends, associates and family, either to change or to remain the same? How can I feel more fulfilled? What parts of myself have gone undeveloped that I would now like to give expression? What faults do I see that I would like to eliminate? What new character traits can I work on developing? How can I set a more realistic goal for the future? What new beliefs can be adopted to replace the delusions of the past?" The possibilities of occupational therapy activities to help with the planning process are endless. Furthermore, the potential for self-discovery and exploration of options are maximized in group treatment.

Individuation at Mid-life

At mid-life, individuation is a continuation of past processes. An increasingly separate existence has been evolving since birth, gradually forming clearer boundaries between the self and the outside world. This individuation plays a part at each transition. Levinson takes his cue from Jung in describing the mid-life individuation tasks as resolving four polarities: young/old, destruction/creation, masculine/feminine and attachment/separateness. Every life structure necessitates giving high priority to certain aspects of the self while minimizing others. In young adulthood, youth, creativity, masculinity and attachment often outweigh their counterparts. At mid-life, neglected parts urgently seek expression.

The Young/Old Polarity Young and old are viewed as relative terms, not specifically tied with any age. Young takes on such meanings as birth, growth, possibility, initiation, openness, energy, potential, promise of spring, fertility and vision of things to come. Conversely, old represents termination, fruition, stability, rigidity, completion, impotence, senility and death.

The issues of the young/old dichotomy at mid-life are realization of one's own death, fear of loss of youth, decline in bodily and psychological powers, realization that one's time is limited, wish for immortality and fear that man is not immortal, loss of omnipotence and acceptance of limitation. Out of the recognition of one's own mortality comes the imagery of the legacy, or what a man will pass on to future generations. Among possible legacies are children, teachings or discoveries, concrete and social structures, objects of lasting value, written documents and artistic works.

The Destruction/Creation Polarity A new awareness of the destruction as a universal process takes on several forms in the mid-life transition. A man must come to an understanding of his grievances toward others for their destructiveness toward him. This typically results in anger toward loved ones: parents, wife, mentors and friends whom he sees as having hurt him. He must also look at his own destructiveness in terms of how he has hurt others. It is necessary for him to accept destructiveness as a natural part of life and to take responsibility for it. Taking action in any direction always has consequences, some creative and some destructive. "If he is forced to maintain the illusion that destructiveness does not exist, he will also be impaired in his capacity for creating, loving and affirming life" (Levinson 1978, 224).

The Masculine/Feminine Polarity Levinson refers to the terms masculine and feminine as going beyond the biological and social differentiation. Masculinity refers to bodily prowess and toughness, homosexuality, rationality, achievement and ambition, and an intolerance of weakness. Femininity refers to motherhood, caring and emotionality, artistic creativity, softness and lack of strength and stamina. The masculine and feminine are really both aspects of the same person, and are seen as poorly integrated in early adulthood, due to immaturity, cultural tradition and the necessity for aggressive pursuit of one's occupation and social position. In middle adulthood, however, man comes to new terms with this polarity, seeing masculine and feminine as less rigidly divided within the self and combining them more creatively in work, personal relationships and acceptance of self. Aggressiveness may give way to a more nurturing and sensitive side of the personality without really injuring the masculine role identity. The resolution of the masculine/ feminine dichotomy opens new possibilities for the man in both love relationships with peer women and mentor relationships.

In occupational therapy, we are constantly faced with the masculine and feminine identities of our patients. In doing activity groups with male and female patients, it is important to consider their values and expectations. For example, male patients, especially those of Hispanic origin, will refuse to do activities like cooking or sewing, which they consider to be "women's work." Female patients may have negative feelings about doing money management or using power tools. In using developmental theory, the age and gender of our patients as well as their disability will determine what activities they are willing to try.

The Attachment/Separateness Polarity Attachment is defined by Levinson as "to be engaged, involved, needy, plugged in, seeking and rooted" (1978, 239). Separateness is distinguished from isolation and loneliness in that it refers to a person's involvement in his inner world, his fantasies. In early adulthood, with marriage and mentor relationships, typically attachment takes precedence at the expense of separateness. At mid-life, developmentally a more equal balance between the two must be achieved. This generally means the man at mid-life moves further into himself, and through this process is able to examine his own feelings, values and goals apart from external and social expectations.

The Late Adult Transition

Levinson positions the late adult transition at ages 60 to 65. The tasks of this period are to reappraise the past, create a new life structure and make choices that are relevant to the final stage of life. Levinson's study does not extend beyond mid-life and must be viewed as speculation. The issues facing the older adult are physical decline, loss of a productive role, and coming to terms with death, both of self and loved ones. According to some theorists, changes in perception of time begin at mid-life, from "time since birth" to "time left to live." In the late adult transition, the approach of death can no longer be ignored. The limited time remaining must be devoted to resolving old conflicts, finishing unfinished business, deepening important relationships and arranging to leave one's legacy. These life tasks lend themselves very nicely to group activities in occupational therapy. Life review groups are one example of how occupational therapy can address these issues.

Physical Decline

By the year 2020, the average life expectancy will be 77 years and 20% of the population in the United States will be over age 65. As people live longer, the effects of normal physical decline become more prominent. At the most basic level, aging cells begin to degenerate and die. Loss of neurons in the brain are the cause of senility and occur naturally, but more rapidly in degenerative diseases like Alzheimer's. Brain cell loss causes functional loss of memory and personality changes as well. Functioning of vital organs, including heart and lungs, slows down. Anatomic changes result in loss of hearing, decline in eyesight, loss of height and lower muscle mass and tone. Most people are familiar with the greying of hair and the general loss of strength and endurance. Osteoporosis or (brittle bones) and osteoarthritis (painful joints) are common.

Changes in the immune system often make older persons more susceptible to disease. Longevity has been shown to be related most closely to heredity. However, regular medical check-ups and a healthy lifestyle are still the best preventive measures. Vulnerability to stress also increases with age. Despite the skills accumulated over a lifetime, change at older ages is still more difficult and more stressful.

Coping with bodily decline requires an acceptance of a more passive role with respect to the environment. Changes in lifestyle which limit physical demands while providing a sense of worth and satisfaction are preferable. Occupational therapy groups can center around energy conservation, setting goals and priorities, exercise and fitness, health education and maintenance and exploring activities that encourage continued use of skills and maintenance of self-esteem and social recognition.

Loss of Productive Role

Retirement may be voluntary or mandatory between ages 60 and 65. Either way, the changes produced by it are many, and show mixed responses in individuals. For some, the increased time to relax and pursue leisure interests is welcome. But for many, retirement is a negative experience that lowers self-worth and leaves them socially isolated. The economic impact of retirement is very real, and those without pensions or retirement plans may find themselves having to accept a lower income and lower socioeconomic status. Retired persons need to find a new structure to replace the work role, and new interests to give them a sense of self-worth. Occupational therapy groups dealing with retirement issues can address time management, financial management, leisure planning, community involvement, volunteering, socialization, new skill development and many others.

Coming to Terms With Death

Loss is a predominant theme in the lives of older people. Erikson's view of the final conflict to be resolved may be helpful in understanding how loss can be accepted. His eighth stage, integrity vs. despair, suggests that contentment in old age results from the view of a life productively lived (Kaplan 1988). The late adult transition necessarily includes reviewing one's life experiences, and reappraising them to sum up their worth. The results of this reappraisal may determine how an individual copes with the later years. At best, in later life grandparents enjoy spoiling their grandchildren and retired workers enjoy knowing that the younger generations will benefit from their life's work. Teachers may enjoy watching the success of their students, for example. According to Erikson, peace and contentment in old age occurs only if one has previously achieved intimacy and generativity. An older person needs to know that his life has been productive and he has passed on his wisdom to others in some way. Without this belief,

157

there is only despair. Despair, according to Erikson, is indicated by a fear of death, and the realization that it's too late to start over.

Preparation for death is another necessary prerequisite of integrity in old age. As life is reappraised, old conflicts and unfinished business may be recalled. It is not unusual to wish for reconciliations with estranged friends or relatives. Often there are old wrongs to be forgiven, apologies to make and unkept promises to be reconsidered. These are important emotional concerns of the elderly, and should not be prematurely dismissed. Those who are physically or cognitively impaired may need help in dealing with these issues. Even when actual reconciliations are not feasible, a great deal can be done through group experiences incorporating role play and other creative activities. Developing a point of view about death is a spiritual and philosophical concern. Carl Rogers, psychotherapist and major spokesman for humanistic psychology, described a new interest in his seventies as he explored the world of the paranormal with his wife. His experiences changed his understanding of death. Whereas in his fifties and sixties he regarded death to be the end of the individual, he now considers it possible that the spiritual essence of man continues to live after death. He mentions the views of Arthur Koestler about each individual's consciousness being a part of the "cosmic consciousness" (Rogers 1980, 88), a view which echoes Jung's ideas regarding the collective unconscious. Zemke and Gratz (1982) point out that for the aged, illness and disability tend to renew earlier crises. "The (occupational) therapist must acknowledge and work toward resolution of these just as she would with any other disabled adult. Only then can the ego integrity crisis be faced. Techniques such as remotivation or life review provide a basis for the thoughtful review and acceptance of life experience necessary for resolution at this final stage of life" (Zemke 1982, 61).

Kohlberg and Wilcox

Kohlberg and Wilcox built on the work of Piaget, who developed stages of intellectual development. They looked at the way logic was used in the development of moral reasoning. How people get along in society, their view of themselves and the social structure depend on how they make decisions about right and wrong. Kohlberg and Wilcox suggest three levels and six stages of moral development (Table 6-4). This perspective is useful in planning groups with patients who are not psychotic, but have problems with society or in dealing with authority figures or rules. Motivation to move up to the next level is having experiences which contradict one's former beliefs, and cause them to question their own reasoning. According to Kohlberg, all of the stages can be brought into adulthood. Many adults have been found to operate at the pre-conventional and conventional levels. Therapists should look for lags in moral reasoning as a possible explanation of behavior in patients (and staff).

Bruce and Borg (1985) suggest that occupational therapy group leaders encourage growth in moral reasoning by creating dissonance. Therapists do this by exposing the group members to reasoning at a slightly higher level, and encouraging role-taking and role-reversal. Introducing moral dilemmas for a group to discuss and problem-solve might provide an appropriate setting for this kind of developmental learning.

Gilligan—"A Different Voice"

Gilligan (1982) challenges previous theories of development in two respects. She sheds doubt on the "age and stage" concept of development, and she suggests that women have a different way of thinking about life than men do and that their developmental stages may also be fundamentally different. Gilligan points out that prior theorists, including Erikson, Kohlberg and Levinson, have based their beliefs primarily on observations of men. A professor at Harvard, Gilligan performed her own research regarding men and women from childhood through maturity, regarding their identity and moral development, rights and responsibilities, and the role of conflict in development.

In relation to Kohlberg, Gilligan suggests that these stages relate more to men than women and do not consider the variables of culture, time, occasion and gender. She observes that events of women's lives and of history promote the view that concern with individual survival is "selfish" or "bad" as opposed to the "responsibility" of a life lived in relationships. For women, life is caring in relationships. When the focus on individuation and individual achievement extends into adulthood and maturity is equated with personal autonomy, concern with relationships appears as a weakness of women rather than a human strength.

The stereotypes of adulthood or maturity suggested by Levinson and Erikson favor separateness or self-sufficiency over connection to others, primarily a "male" point of view, according to Gilligan. According to these theorists, young adulthood is characterized by a conflict of commitment in which either identity or intimacy wins out. The male believes that separation empowers the self and permits full self-expression; intimacy, the choice of women, represents immaturity and impedes expression of the self. Gilligan states that "the silence of women in the narrative of adult development distorts the conception of its stages and sequence" (Gilligan 1982, 156).

Gilligan does not suggest an alternative sequence of developmental stages, nor does she describe how pre-established stages are different for women. Yet her points are well-taken, and encourage us, in using this frame of reference, not to accept the proposed ages and stages as absolute reality.

Table 6-4.
Kohlberg and Wilcox Development of Moral Reasoning

Age	Stage
2-4	**Preconventional level: decisions made on the basis of punishment and reward** Stage 1 - person is egocentric — no ablity to empathize Stage 2 - reciprocity — makes deals with authority
6+	**Conventional level: decisions based on pleasing others** Stage 3 - confirms identity as good — authority is fair — good people get best treatment Stage 4 - law and order orientation — rules necessary to maintain social structure — only one system is "right"
11-12	**Post-conventional level: fairness is free standing logic** Stage 5 - individual rights and human dignity can override rules — empathy influences decisions — right and wrong is separate from rules Stage 6 - ideal stage, rarely encountered in reality — unconditional value of rights of humanity — empathized with all participants in a moral dilemma — creatively resolves polarities and contradictions

In considering Gilligan's message for occupational therapy groups, we need to consider more carefully the role of relationships for our patients. There is no better place than a group to explore and work on the skills that affect relationships.

Function and Dysfunction

If one uses an age and stage theory, then healthy functioning is having achieved the appropriate developmental tasks for his age. For example, a 23-year-old will have separated from his parents, chosen a career and if not married, at least developed a support system of peers with whom to identify. Conversely, dysfunction may be looked at as failure to develop age appropriate skills, a failure to achieve the tasks of an age-appropriate stage. The stages of childhood and adolescence have been studied historically in much greater detail than those of adulthood. So as Gilligan implies, it is better to use the ages given for developmental tasks as approximate guidelines. Furthermore, as illness interferes with normal development, the discrepancy between age and developmental level may be so great that the term "age-appropriate" becomes meaningless. It is the developmental stage that we as occupational therapists are concerned with, since that is what determines the level of function and adaptation to the environment. Dysfunction can be seen as a lack of adaptive skills necessary for effective and satisfying interaction with one's environment. It can be caused by a failure to develop these skills (developmental delay), a loss of these skills (due to brain trauma for example), or a regression to an earlier stage of development (such as that caused by depression or schizophrenia).

In adult development theory, just the normal tasks at each transitional stage may be enough to cause a crisis situation. If Levinson speaks of the mid-life transition as a potential crisis for 80% of the population, think of the impact it must have on those with physical or mental disability. If Levinson is right, the stress produced by this kind of crisis is likely to contribute to physical and mental breakdown, even in those without previous illness.

Development is almost always affected by illness. As disabled patients are referred to occupational therapy, the assessment process is likely to uncover missing skills that patients have failed to learn in earlier stages of development. The difficulty in coping with illness in the present is often due to the inadequacy of earlier skill development. Because the stages of development are hierarchical, occupational therapy cannot address issues of the patient's current age until earlier skills are learned. For example, a 20-year-old may not be expected to work on career choice and separation from parents if his or her illness has resulted in a lack of ability to form peer relationships and his own identity is not developed. Because of discrepancies between chronological and developmental age in persons with illness and disability, groups in occupational therapy often include patients of varying ages. Occupational therapists organize treatment groups by developmental levels (not age levels), so that members can work together on similar skills.

Change and Motivation

Motivation comes from an individual's natural desire for mastery of age-appropriate skills. The drive toward mastery is, at least in part, biologically determined. However, as a person matures, the environment plays a greater part in motivation. If a person's attempts to progress developmentally are met with success, motivation will likely remain intact. Repeated failures to keep up with peers, on the other hand, may discourage a person from continuing to try. Occupational therapy may encourage the rediscovery of the drive toward mastery by creating a "just right challenge." This is a task or situation that encourages a patient to use higher level skills, but one that is not beyond his or her reach.

When there is a developmental lag or loss of skills, they must be learned or relearned in the correct developmental sequence. Mosey called this "recapitulation of ontogeny" (Mosey 1970). If the patient is more than one level behind, the change process may be slow, but it follows a more or less predictable pattern. Since developmental stages are hierarchical, the earlier skills must be mastered before the learning of later developing skills is possible.

Consider a group of individuals with chronic mental illness. The age of onset for several chronic mental illnesses is the early 20s. Often patients have achieved at least some of the developmental tasks of the young adult transition before becoming ill. Many have vocational or educational training in a chosen career, some have begun working and have moved out of their parents' homes, some have married and had one or two children. These are accomplishments beyond the capacity of most patients with chronic mental illness. One might see these patients as regressed. Because of their illness, they have gone backward to an earlier, less mature stage of development. In treating these patients, the occupational therapist needs to determine the correct level at which to begin. This will be the level at which mastery is possible and growth and change can be motivated.

Mosey's concept of the six adaptive skills is helpful in identifying a patient's correct developmental level, as well as determining which skills need work. These skills are: perceptual-motor, cognitive, dyadic interaction, group interaction, self-identity and sexual identity skills. Each adaptive skill has several subskills whose typical ages of development are identified. These are described fully in her text, *Psychosocial Components of Occupational Therapy* (1986) (see Appendix C).

Change occurs through the learning of new skills. This can be encouraged by setting up a growth-facilitating environment. The occupational therapist looks carefully at the physical environment in terms of safety. The emotional environment may best be set through the patient-therapist relationship and through the use of groups. Mosey's concept of the developmental groups is useful here. The hierarchy of group structure and leadership requirements in these groups can help occupational therapists to plan treatment groups for patients that are appropriate to their level of development (see Appendix B).

However, the benefits of group treatment go beyond the learning or re-learning of group interaction skill. All six adaptive skills identified by Mosey may be effectively learned in a group context through occupational therapy activity. At the higher developmental levels, the tasks of adult development may be facilitated through group activities in occupational therapy.

Group Treatment

It has been implied that groups in this frame of reference are best organized along the lines of developmental level. Occupational therapy groups would be primarily homogeneous. At lower levels, patients in a parallel group may be participating in activities that promote sensorimotor or cognitive skill development. At higher levels, groups may use interaction skills to work on career choice in the young adult transition, re-examine their values in the mid-life transition, or participate in retirement planning in the late life transition. The structure of occupational therapy treatment groups is organized according to the developmental level, and this guides the occupational therapist's choice of activity as well.

The limitations for use of this frame of reference are minimal. Patients of every age and almost any type of disability are appropriately treated within its bounds. The theories of adult development described in this chapter, however, are most helpful in planning groups for the later stages of development. Guidelines for the earlier stages, dealing with sensorimotor and cognitive development, are described in Chapter 7.

Role of the Leader

In developmental groups, the occupational therapist takes a directive role. Knowledge of the predictable conflicts and skills in each developmental stage guides the use of activities and setting of group goals. He/she evaluates patients' skills to determine their developmental levels, and attempts to predict their potential for further development. When placed in appropriate groups, patients can work together on their mutual tasks with the leader's guidance. Because the sequence of learned tasks is hierarchical, the occupational therapist cannot give too many choices to the group. If the groups are planned appropriately, their area of interest should coincide with the developmental tasks of their level. Occupational therapists need to challenge their groups to develop further by consistently introducing higher level activities at appropriate times.

It is also the responsibility of the leader to create and maintain a growth facilitating environment (Mosey 1970). In the treatment setting, patients should be supported and rewarded for growth, not discouraged. If a group is ready to take on more responsibility, this should be allowed. If growing requires a stage of upset and turmoil, and it has to get worse before it gets better, this should also be met with patience and support.

The occupational therapist should be on the lookout for signs of developmental transitions in patients with physical disability as well as mental illness. Even when the illness is physical, addressing developmental issues can be the most beneficial in helping the patient to cope. Coping with illness or developmental crises often requires the learning of enabling skills. These are specific cognitive, psychosocial or sensorimotor learned behaviors that make it possible for the individual to meet his developmental needs (Bruce and Borg 1987). Examples are reading and writing, communication skills or the ability to empathize with others. Mosey's adaptive skills might be used as a guide.

Examples of Activities

Those activities chosen should address issues to be resolved or specific skills appropriate to the developmental level of the patient group. The theorist, the specific stage to be addressed and the specific task or skill within that stage should be identified. Since most of the theorists have an identified hierarchy of issues, tasks or skills to be learned at each level, these can easily serve as guidelines for activity choice. Here are some examples.

Ideal Man/Ideal Woman

This activity addresses Levinson's early adult transition, specifically, the tasks of finding a special woman or man, and finding a mentor.

Materials: 12"x18" sheets of white drawing paper, pastels, pencils, erasers and kleenex

Directions: First look into your fantasy, and envision a person of the opposite sex whom you consider to be ideal, having all the qualities you would wish for in a mate, companion and friend. What does that person look like? Notice hair, eyes, facial expression, stature, clothing, style of movement. What is that person doing? Perhaps he or she is sitting across from you at dinner, participating with you in an active sport, sitting by the fireside planning a new project with you, having lively interactions with others at a party, seriously engaging in a business venture or walking alone on a deserted beach. When an image has come to mind, try to capture its essential qualities by drawing them.

Fold the paper in half and draw your first picture on the left half of the page. Never mind if your drawing doesn't look exactly like your mental image - just do the best that you can. You have 15 minutes for the drawing. After ten minutes, next to your drawing make note of any particular personality traits, habits, attitudes, values and other internal attributes possessed by the person you drew. Is this person sensitive, strong, energetic, intellectual, responsible, gentle? What talents and abilities does the person possess? Now imagine a person of the same sex, whom you consider to be ideal. Maybe the person is someone whose accomplishments you admire or whose lifestyle seems appealing. Perhaps the person holds a position in life you aspire to, or has talents you desire to develop in yourself. Do not think too much about this, but allow images to enter your mind, remembering that this will be a person you create, not necessarily someone you know. You may combine attributes of several people or just make up new ones. Keep in mind the images you consider most ideal and when the image crystallizes, begin to draw it on the second side of your paper. Do the same as you did for the first part, considering physical appearance, activity or situation, and both external and internal traits. Write down those elements which cannot be defined by drawing (15 minutes).

Times of Your Life Collage

This activity addresses Levinson's mid-life transition in providing an opportunity to review past accomplishments as well as unrealized expectations. It will assist patients in re-evaluating the past and present life structures in preparation for making changes in middle adulthood (Figure 6-1).

Materials: Variety of magazines suitable to patients, large poster board, glue, scissors and marker for each patient. Posterboard may be set up ahead of time to provide a space for each five years of their life up to their present age. If patients in the group are of similar or known ages, this may be done ahead of time by the therapist as follows. Example, for patient age 40:

Directions: the object of this exercise is to get a temporal perspective on our lives, and to see how the parts fit into the whole to make us the people we are today. The posterboard will represent the whole. Our life will begin on the upper left and proceed to the lower right, divided into time intervals of five years. Leave one space for the present. (Therapist should show example.) Now think about the events that occurred in each segment of your life, what you were like then, people who were in your life then, places where you lived or traveled, accomplishments you made, decisions you made. Then look through the magazines and find pictures, words and phrases that best describe the major event or aspect of each segment of your life up to and including the present.

0-5	5-10	10-15	15-20
20-25	25-30	3-35	35-40

Figure 6-1. Times of your life collage.

This activity can take up to two hours. Depending on patient group, the project can be done on one day, discussed the next, or it can carry over several group sessions. Discussion should center around evaluation of events and account for spaces left blank. High and low points may be identified. Emotional responses to events or patterns may be identified. Are there patterns? Were there changes? How were the changes made? Markers may be used to identify highs, lows, emotions surrounding events.

Change options should then be explored. What accounts for the decisions in your life? Were they made impulsively? Influenced by others? Done with careful planning? If you could go back and change parts of your life, what would you change? What do you wish you could add or delete? What was missing in your life development that you wish had been there?

A follow-up drawing can be added to this exercise, entitled "the future." Planning the next five or ten years can be done, using the same collage techniques.

Fabric of Life

This simple weaving activity addresses the life review task of the Levinson's late adult transition. It is in keeping with the views of Erikson and Jung as well. The use of colors, patterns and materials encourage the incorporation of emotional as well as substantive memories, or essences as well as marker events (Figure 6-2.). This exercise requires two or three one-hour sessions for most groups.

Materials: Pencils and paper, and a medium paper bag for each group member to plan his/her project. A heavy wire circle (loom) 12"-18" in diameter (warped with strong yarn dividing the circle into 16 equal parts, tied together in the center), and one pair of sharp scissors should be provided for each person. A large variety of fabric remnants (can be scraps from a seamstress or cut from old, donated clothes, curtains, sheets, tablecloths etc.), trimmings, ribbons and several colored balls of yarn. Fabrics should be cut into long 1" strips.

Directions: Fabrics are, for most of us, associated with clothing, home furnishings, draperies, bed sheets, and the like. They are adorning and surrounding us constantly, and although often not the focus of our attention, they influence our sensory experiences and our mood and color our lives in ways of which we may be unaware.

In this exercise, we will associate key events, places and persons in our lives with a sensory awareness of the fabrics that may symbolize them. We will choose fabrics, trimmings or ribbons to represent both events and significant others in our lives. In

Figure 6-2. Fabric of life.

addition, each of us will choose one special yarn or fabric to represent ourselves. Begin by writing down any of the following which apply most to you. As you choose fabrics, trimmings and ribbons for each memory, cut an arm's length of it and place it in your paper bag.

1. Birth and young childhood - envision your room or most memorable environment as a child. What do you see? What can you feel? Is there a favorite blanket or stuffed toy? What color is there? How does the texture of the fabric feel to your touch? Choose a fabric or material from the collection to represent this association as closely as possible.

2. Parents - envision each of your parents, either separately or together, doing whatever they ordinarily were doing when you were a child. How were they dressed? What was their favorite color, style? Summon an image of each of your parents as you would like to remember them from childhood. Then choose a fabric to represent that image.

Take a few minutes to re-experience visual, tactile, auditory or olfactory memories (sights, sounds, textures and smells) associated with each of the items to follow, and continue to select fabrics and place them in your bag.

3. Friends from childhood
4. Relatives and siblings
5. A childhood home - imagine your room
6. First day of school - what did you wear?

  7. Communion, bar mitzvah, or joining a church
  8. First date
  9. First school dance
 10. First boyfriend or girlfriend
 11. Graduation
 12. First job (or significant ones)
 13. Marriage
 14. First house or apartment
 15. Death of loved one(s)
 16. Important travels
 17. Awards or promotions at work
 18. Adult friends
 19. Birth of children and their significant others
 20. Marriage, graduation or jobs of children
 21. Birth of grandchildren
 22. Organizations or committees
 23. Adult hobbies, leisure activities
 24. Other important events or milestones

Planning takes at least a one-hour session, and should be discussed before the session ends. Memories can be verbalized and elaborated. If desired, a small scrap of fabric can be taped to the paper and labeled after each item planned, so the group member won't forget which was chosen for which at the next session. Be sure to put names on paper bags. Planning paper can be folded and placed inside.

Procedure for weaving: Begin with the ball of yarn that represents you. Tie the end to the center and weave it under and over each warp thread, clockwise around the circle for five or six rows. This yarn will touch and become a part of all the other materials you have chosen. How much of each other material you use depends on how large a part its associated element played in your life. Begin with childhood and work chronologically, adding chosen materials and weaving them over and under with the yarn, around and around the circle. From time to time, rake the yarn toward the center with your fingers to push it together. End when you have used up all the materials selected. Wind the yarn (or add ribbon or trim) around and around the wire circle to cover it, and tie in a loop knot at the end to hang it on the wall.

Discussion should be encouraged during the weaving process, and the therapist will help patients as needed. Feelings about the project at the end are especially important. The doing process often evokes many hidden feelings that need to be expressed and explored. Is the review of life positive or negative? Which parts are positive or negative? What is missing? Patients should be encouraged to keep their own projects and to reflect on the significance of them, and not to use them as gifts, at least for awhile. Remember, a life review is only the beginning of the task of evaluation and integration which Jung and Erikson have suggested is necessary for contentment in old age.

The Doctor's Dilemma

This activity refers to Kohlberg's fourth and fifth stages of moral development. The group's discussion is intended to cast doubt upon a strict "law and order" kind of reasoning about morality, and to encourage empathy with more than one participant in a given situation.

Materials: none

Directions: First I will read you a story which has several characters who do not agree with one another. Listen carefully to the story and then, as a group, decide who is right, who is wrong, and what should be done about the situation.

Story: The Doctor's Dilemma

Jenny was a young, healthy 24-year-old woman who went into the hospital unexpectedly to have her appendix removed. It was 8:00 pm and Dr. Strothers had just completed a long tiring day of surgery. Jenny's sister Carol brought her to the hospital in terrible pain; it was evident that she needed to be operated on at once. The emergency room nurse, Eva, interviewed Jenny and prepared her for surgery. Eva wrote down on her report that Jenny had her last meal one hour ago, which put her at considerable risk of choking when given general anesthesia. However, the doctor did not read the report carefully. He operated anyway, and the patient choked to death on the table.

Carol was in shock; she suspected negligence and sued the doctor for one million dollars. Although Jenny was not married and had no children, Carol missed her sister and felt that those who mistreated her sister should pay. But mostly, she could really use the money. She and her husband had just bought a house, and had defaulted on the last few payments. Five hundred thousand dollars would just about pay off their mortgage, and prevent them from losing their home.

Eva, the nurse who prepared the report, was secretly in love with the doctor. Out of love, she offered to alter the report, changing the "one" hour since last meal to a "nine." This would clear Dr. Strothers of any blame for Jenny's death. Eva saw that Dr. Strothers was a caring and brilliant young doctor, capable of saving many more lives if allowed to continue his practice. Of course, a verdict of guilty in the lawsuit would prevent him from ever practicing again. Eva was willing to give up nursing and take the blame for the man she loved. She hoped perhaps he would marry her if she did this, and after a brief jail sentence, they could live happily ever after.

Dr. Strothers was faced with a dilemma. Should he take the blame, plead guilty in the lawsuit, and give up his life's work? Should he accept Eva's offer to take the blame? Should he meet with Carol and offer to pay her five hundred thousand dollars to withdraw the lawsuit? How should the story end? It's up to you.

Group Leadership

The seven stages of groups can remain intact when working with most adult groups in this frame of reference. The introduction is done according to the guidelines offered in Chapter 1.

Activity

Activities and goals are chosen using specific guidelines from the ages and stages of development. The learning exercise in Table 6-5 may be helpful in identifying the theory and stage which is appropriate for your particular patients. Fill in the chart by writing under the various chronological ages the appropriate information from the theories reviewed at the beginning of this chapter.

It is especially important to plan an environment that incorporates safety, support and challenge. The goals for these groups are to help members progress to higher levels of development. The timing of groups may be altered to suit the group, the activity and the goal. Many of the tasks of adult development are quite complex, and there are many aspects to be explored. Activities such as those listed above may take several sessions, depending on how they are planned and how much discussion seems appropriate. If patients are motivated by a particular activity, it may be desirable to give homework. Patients may be asked to think about the issues discussed between sessions, to explore options for change or to try out new behaviors with family and friends.

Sharing and Processing

Sharing, including self-expression and feedback, are important parts of the developmental group. However, while members are working on similar tasks, there is no expectation that they will produce similar results, since each person must complete a developmental task in his own way.

Processing the group may uncover many feelings about both past and present experience. This is one frame of reference in which talking about past events is not discouraged. Relationships among members evidenced during processing can be helpful in supporting patients through many traumatic memories as well as stressful present day realities. Group cohesiveness in this frame is desirable and encouraged.

Generalizing and Application

Generalizing an experience should be somewhat predictable, since most of the activities will address specific developmental issues. The therapist really has to take the lead, to guide the discussion of general principles along developmental lines.

Application is a particularly important aspect of developmental groups, since the group experiences are designed to have a specific impact on development. If there is a focus to the discussion of developmental groups, it should be the application of learning to each individual's everyday life. The summary can be shared by members and leader, depending on the ability of the group, and this should also stress application of learning.

Table 6-5.
Developmental Theories Comparitive Chart

Directions: Using information from this text and others, fill in the developmental stages for each of the latest theorists.

Chronological Age	0-1	2	5	10	15	20	25	30	40	45	50	60	65
Jung Spiritual Stages													
Erikson Psychosocial Stages													
Levinson Life Transitions													
Kohlberg Moral Development													
Mosey Adaptive Skills													
Sensory Integrative Cognitive													
Dyadic Interaction Group Interaction													
Self Identity Sexual Identity													
Physical Milestones													

Bibliography

Bruce MA. and Borg B. *Frames of Reference in Psychosocial Occupational Therapy*, Thorofare, NJ: SLACK Inc., 1987.

Cole, M. and Gross, M. *Structured Group Experiences for Life's Adult Transitions*, 1982, unpublished.

Gilligan C. *A Different Voice*, Cambridge MA: Harvard University Press, 1982.

Kaplan H. and Sadock B. *Synopsis of Psychiatry*. 6th ed. Baltimore: Williams & Wilkins, 1991.

Levinson D. *The Seasons of a Man's Life*, NY: Ballentine Books, 1978.

Mosey AC. *Three Frames of Reference for Mental Health*. Thorofare NJ: SLACK Inc., 1970.

Mosey AC. *Psychosocial Components of Occupational Therapy*. New York, Raven, 1986.

Rogers C. *A Way of Being*. Boston: Houghton Mifflin, 1980.

Schultz D. *Theories of Personality*. Monterrey, CA: Brooks/Cole, 1976.

Sheehy G. *Passages: Predictable Crises of Adult Life*. NY: EP Dutton, 1974.

Viorst J. *Necessary Losses*. NY: Ballentine Books, 1986.

Wilcox M. *Developmental Journey*. Nashville: Abbington Press, 1979.

Zemke R. and Gratz RR. The Role of Theory: Erikson and Occupational Therapy, *Occupational Therapy in Mental Health*, 1982, II, 3, 45-63.

Chapter

7

A Neurodevelopmental Approach

The neurodevelopmental approach is being used as a broad category which addresses sensorimotor, perceptual and cognitive problems due to brain dysfunction. Treatment in this frame, according to Trombly (1989), is aimed at promoting re-development of these abilities based on principles of neurophysiology. "When the treatment of these losses follows a developmental sequence and techniques reflect anatomical, functional or behavioral reorganization in the central nervous system, the approach is called **neuro-developmental**"(Trombly 1989, 39). For occupational therapy, the primary use of this frame of reference has been with developmental disabilities affecting the central nervous system and those who have suffered trauma or disease to the central nervous system. However, recent studies of the brain have linked neurophysiological abnormalities and central nervous system dysfunction to mental disorders as well. Applying neurodevelopmental principles of treatment with the geriatric population is increasing and shows promising results. Occupational therapy groups using this frame of reference should use activities that stimulate the senses, produce purposeful movement, promote cognition and affect the central nervous system in a systematic way.

Basic Assumptions

This frame of reference encompasses many theorists (and techniques), among them Rood, Bobath, Brunnstrom and Ayres and proprioceptive neuromuscular facilitation (PNF). These approaches are not necessarily intended to be used with groups, however, the principles of treatment can be applied when planning group activities. Examples of occupational therapy group treatment approaches using these theories are reviewed, including the writings of King, Ross and Levy. Central to all of these approaches is the assumption that rehabilitation of perceptual, sensorimotor and cognitive disorders follows a developmental sequence. All of the theorists agree on the importance of sensation in this process, and the importance of repetition to learning. Disagreement centers around the focus of conscious attention. Rood, the Bobaths and Ayres believe the focus should be on the goal of movement, rather than the movement itself. There is also disagreement about the role of primitive reflexes. Brunnstrom fosters the conscious use of reflexes to elicit movement in the disabled adult, while the Bobath approach actively inhibits reflexes (Trombly 1979).

Rood

Margaret Rood's work preceded most of the other theorists covered in this chapter, and her ideas seem to have inspired many of the concepts of sensory integration developed later. Rood was the first to focus on the importance of reflexes. She states "motor patterns are developed from fundamental reflex patterns present at birth which are utilized and gradually modified through sensory stimuli until the highest control is gained on the conscious cortical level. It seemed to me then, that if it were possible to apply the proper sensory stimuli to the appropriate sensory receptor as it is utilized in normal sequential development, it might be possible to elicit motor responses reflexly and by following neurophysiological principles, establish proper motor engrams"(Rood 1954). Rood's theory has four basic components: 1) sensory input is required for normalization of tone and evocation of desired muscular responses, 2) sensorimotor control is developmentally based, 3) movement is purposeful and 4) repetition of movement is necessary for learning.

Most occupational therapists recognize Rood's techniques of facilitation and inhibition. Light stroking, brushing, icing and joint compression are used to facilitate movement. Joint approximation (light compression), neutral warmth, pressure on tendon insertion and slow rhythmical movement are used to inhibit unwanted movement. Rood recommended the facilitation of normal movement in a developmental sequence. First, phasic reciprocal contraction, such as flexion to extension and back, are practiced repeatedly until learned. Next, stabilization through co-contraction of major muscle groups is facilitated. A third phase combines these, practicing movement imposed on stabilization, and a final phase incorporates the development of skilled movement.

This early theorist identified eight ontogenetic motor patterns as follows:
1. supine withdrawal
2. segmental rolling
3. pivot prone (prone extension)
4. neck co-contraction
5. supporting self on elbows
6. all fours movement patterns
7. standing
8. walking

This sequence gives occupational therapists some very specific guidelines for planning movement activities for patients with neurodevelopmental disorders. When planning group treatment, each patient's unique developmental level with respect to movement needs to be carefully considered. Movement groups can be set up at many levels, but should progress from earlier to later stages in the ontogenetic sequence. Patients should not be asked to perform movements at higher levels than they are capable. Positioning is a primary concern, especially at the lower levels. It may involve the extensive use of mats, bolsters, beach balls or other specialized equipment.

Many games can be devised that involve pushing and pulling, throwing and catching, rolling and creeping to move the body from one place to another. These activities should be set up to incorporate the correct therapeutic movement sequences for each patient, while the patients are participating in goal-directed activities.

The Bobaths

Dr. and Mrs. Bobath are a neurologist and a physiotherapist from England who originated the therapeutic technique best known as "neuro-developmental therapy" (NDT) (Bobath 1972). One of their most important contributions to theory is their focus on sensorimotor learning. It is not movement itself, but the sensation of movement that is learned and remembered. Much of the Bobaths' work was done on children with cerebral palsy and adult stroke patients. The techniques are widely known and used, but little researched, according to Trombly (1989). Following their focus on sensation, their handling of children with cerebral palsy and subsequently of adults with hemiplegia, concentrated on repetition of correct motor responses. The assumption is that when patients experience normal movement, this results in correct sensory feedback to the central nervous system. Neurodevelopmental therapy involves teaching the patient how correct movement feels (Trombly 1989). To this end, great effort is made to inhibit primitive reflexes through "reflex inhibiting patterns"(RIP's) (Trombly 1989, 113), and to elicit righting and equilibrium responses.

In NDT, sensory stimulation is regulated with great care. Weight bearing, placing and holding, tapping and joint compression are used to activate normal movement and posture. However, these stimuli are withdrawn as soon as an abnormal response occurs. In hemiplegia, sensory deficits are interpreted as an indication of poor prognosis for regaining normal control of movement. Stress is avoided, since it is thought to promote abnormal tone and movement.

After stroke or head trauma, the sequence of re-learning movement approximates normal development. Compensatory movement such as practicing dressing or feeding is discouraged because it results in increased spasticity and inactivity of the involved side. Recovery from stroke and trauma generally involves a flaccid stage followed by a spastic stage. Many specific exercises and handling are suggested in each of these stages following the developmental process. These involve positioning, weight bearing, holding and placing, balance reactions and protective extension, among others. Trombly (1989) suggests a good source of both individual and group activities based on the Bobath NDT approach is Egger's *Occupational Therapy in the Treatment of Adult Hemiplegia* (1983).

Brunnstrom

Unlike the other theorists so far, Signe Brunnstrom took an opposite view of the use of reflexes. Her basic assumption was that as normal development progresses, spinal cord and brain stem reflexes become modified and their components rearranged into purposeful movement through the central nervous system. Therefore reflexes can and *should* be used to elicit movement where none exists as part of a normal sequence (Trombly 1989). Both proprioceptive (resistive) and exteroceptive (tactile) stimuli are used to elicit reflexes, and the patient is encouraged to think about the movement that results and try to gain control of that movement.

The Brunnstrom approach seeks to elicit associated reactions and synergies. Resistive stimuli are believed to achieve both reflexive movement on the non-involved side, for example, and similar synergistic movement on the involved side. A **synergy** is defined as the total flexion or extension movement of a joint or limb.

Six stages of recovery are defined by Brunnstrom for the upper and lower extremity. Generally these are:

1. flaccidity, no voluntary movement
2. synergies or minimal voluntary movement
3. synergies performed voluntarily
4. some deviation from synergy
5. independent or isolated movement
6. individual joint movement nearly normal with minimal spasticity.

These are specifically defined, and interested students are encouraged to read about specific assessment and treatment techniques in Brunnstrom's *Movement Therapy in Hemiplegia* (1970).

Proprioceptive Neuromuscular Facilitation

The PNF approach, developed by neurophysiologist Herman Kabat, PhD MD, uses proprioceptor stimulation to hasten the response and recovery of neuromuscular mechanisms. The theory has been developing since the early 1940s, and has had many esteemed contributors, including Sherrington, Gessell and Pavlov. Diagonal and spiraling patterns of movement were identified to parallel functional movement such as that used in sports.

PNF literature states eleven basic principles (Trombly 1989):

1. All human beings have potentials that are not fully developed.
2. Normal motor development proceeds in a cervico-caudal and proximodistal direction.
3. Early motor learning is dominated by reflex activity. Mature motor behavior is reinforced or supported by postural reflex mechanisms.
4. The growth of motor behavior has cyclic trends as evidenced by shifts between flexor and extensor dominance.
5. Goal-directed activity is made up of reversing movements.
6. Normal movement and posture are dependent upon "synergism" and a balanced interaction of antagonists.
7. Developing motor behavior is expressed in an orderly sequence of total patterns of movement and posture.
8. Normal motor development has an orderly sequence but lacks a step-by-step quality. Overlapping occurs.
9. Improvement of motor ability is dependent upon motor learning.
10. Frequency of stimulation and repetition of activity are used to promote retention of motor learning and the development of strength and endurance.
11. Goal-directed activities, coupled with techniques of facilitation, are used to hasten learning of total patterns of walking and of self-care activities.

The PNF techniques involve two diagonal patterns of movement for every major part of the body: head, neck, trunk and extremities. These patterns combine the simplest movements: abduction, adduction, internal/external rotation and crossing the midline. The patterns are unilateral and bilateral, symmetrical and assymetrical, and total body movements. All functional movements are related to these patterns, which are learned and relearned through repetition. The techniques are similar to Brunnstrom in that they encourage the patient to think about the movement and assist the therapist, often using auditory commands: "Look up! Swing down! Help me move you!" (Trombly 1989). These techniques are specifically described in Trombly (1989), and the interested student is referred to this text for a more in-depth description.

Groups using the principles of PNF as well as other neurodevelopmental theories may be designed with patients who have achieved a fair degree of voluntary movement. Exercise groups, movement to music, and simple games are best suited to these patients, many of whom are likely to have language and cognitive problems as well.

Ayres

A. Jean Ayres is best known for her contributions to the theory of sensory integration. This approach assumes that the central nervous system organizes and integrates sensory stimuli to produce an adaptive response. Ayres refers to the normal developmental sequence in her study of the use of sensory input. She suggests four levels of the sensory integrative process.

Primary level

At this level Ayres identifies the three basic sensory systems as vestibular, proprioceptive and tactile. Visual and auditory are acknowledged but not thought to play a major integrative role in this early stage. Touch is cited as the basis for the infant's first emotional bond with mother. The processing of these initial touch sensations is seen to be responsible for establishing a basic sense of security.

The proprioceptive and vestibular senses offer another kind of basic security: gravitational security. These help the child develop balance for standing and walking, and prevents the fear of falling. This level includes the eye movements, posture, balance, muscle tone and gravitational security all resulting from the vestibular and proprioceptive integration. Sucking, eating, the mother-child bond and tactile comfort are seen as the result of integration of tactile sensations.

Second level

At this level the three basic senses are integrated into a body **precept**, coordination of the two sides of the body, motor planning, attention span, activity level and emotional stability. Sensory information from vestibular, proprioceptive and tactile receptors are used to form precepts, or maps of the body which are stored in the brain. With this mechanism, one is constantly aware of where his body is and what it is doing. This precept has information about right and left sides of the body, which allow the two sides to work bilaterally to accomplish tasks. The precept also allows a person to plan motor actions, i.e., catching a ball or feeding himself. The organization of sensory input by the brain is also reflected in the ability to focus attention and adjust the level or pace of activity. Hyperactivity and hypoactivity and the inability to attend are thus explained by poor integration at the secondary level of sensory integration.

Third level

Speech and language, eye-hand coordination, visual perception and purposeful activity are possible at this level due to the impact of auditory and visual sensations. According to Ayres, the vestibular and auditory systems are intimately related. The vestibular system, as stated above, is responsible for the ability to attend to what is heard. Language comprehension likewise begins with the child's touching, moving, lifting and otherwise interacting with the objects in his environment. Only through this experience can he begin to appreciate the unique properties of an object and know its name. Visual perception is also seen as an end product of earlier sensory integration: how big something is, how far away it is, and what its relationship is to other parts of the environment are all experienced first by reaching and touching. The visual experience is thus intimately related to the tactile and vestibular systems as well. With an understanding of what he hears and what he sees, the child's actions with respect to the environment can be purposeful. Visual sensation directs the child's hand to reach out to pet the kitten. He alters his posture to keep his balance as the kitten moves under his touch. The child hears the kitten purr and repeats the action. Visual, auditory, tactile and vestibular systems all work together to help the child explore and learn about his environment.

Fourth level

The fourth and final level of sensory integration includes the following end products: the ability to organize and concentrate, self-esteem, control and confidence, academic learning ability, capacity for abstract thought and reasoning and development of dominance and hemispheric specialization. From Ayres' point of view, it does little good for occupational therapists to attempt to directly teach these skills when the earlier stages of integration are not adequately developed.

Skilled voluntary fine motor hand movement, for example, cannot be taught to the disabled child by giving practice exercises. Ayres describes the development of hand movement as a sequence of many steps:
  a. control of neck and eye movements
  b. trunk stability and balance
  c. scapular and shoulder stability and movement
  d. elbow motion
  e. gross grasp
  f. wrist positioning and movement
  g. release of grasp
  h. forearm supination and pronation
  i. individual finger manipulation

Overlapping this sequence is the coordination of visual and sensorimotor mechanisms. Movements begin as spinal reflexes and are modified and refined to achieve a behavioral goal. In this way, reflex movement becomes voluntary. Regarding the role of sensation in this process, Ayres states two basic assumptions: 1) "reflex movements (which) are the precursor to and the foundation of voluntary movement ... are elicited by sensory stimuli," and 2) "ongoing motor learning and behavior are strongly influenced by if not dependent on incoming sensation" (Ayres 1976). She further reflects that although reflex movement can be elicited by direct stimulation, voluntary movement must be **purposeful**. A great deal has been written about sensory integrative function, and the reader is referred to A. Jean Ayre's *The Development of Sensory Integrative Theory and Practice* and *Sensory Integration and the Child* for a more in-depth discussion (Figure 7-1). An updated version of sensory integration theory by Fisher, Murray and Bundy is entitled *Sensory Integration: Theory and Practice* (1991).

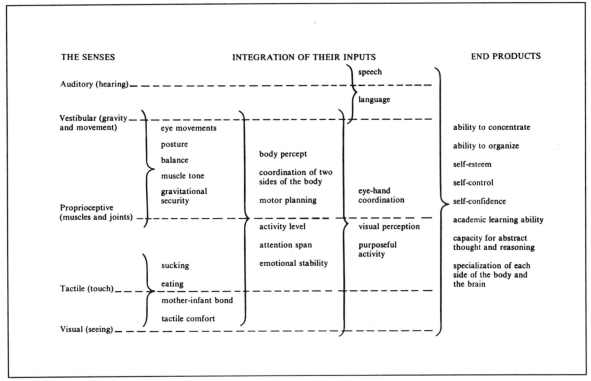

Figure 7-1. A. Jean Ayres sensory integration theory. Reprinted from *Sensory Integration and the Child. (p. 60)* © 1979 by Western Psychological Services, 12031 Wilshire Blvd., Los Angeles, CA 90025.

Group Approaches

King

While most of the research of Ayres and her associates applies to children, several occupational therapists have written about the treatment of mentally ill adults using neurodevelopmental and sensory integrative techniques. The best known of these is Lorna Jean King, who pioneered the use of sensory integration approaches with chronic schizophrenic adults.

Lorna Jean King has noted the lack of sensory integration in both schizophrenic and autistic patients by observing the kinds of sensory stimulation they seek from the environment. For example, she evaluates a retarded and autistic adolescent by observing his preference for vibratory input (plays with a hand held vibrator), proprioceptive input (constant self-hugging) and calming vestibular input (distractable and disruptive behavior is reduced by slow swinging and rocking) (Larrington 1987).

Paul Schilder noted as early as the 1930s that schizophrenic patients are markedly under-reactive to vestibular stimulation as measured by **postrotary nystagmus,** (rapid eye movements) (King 1974). King linked the vestibular system abnormalities with the postural and movement limitations (pacing, adduction and internal rotation) observed in the chronic process schizophrenic patient, more currently called the negative symptom schizophrenic (Figure 7-2). **Process schizophrenia** is a subtype of schizophrenia, a mental

Figure 7-2. Postural abnormalities due to faulty proprioceptive feedback in the person with process schizophrenia. (flexion, adduction, internal rotation).

disorder which develops insidiously from childhood and is not the result of a severe or recognizable stress. Process schizophrenics do not respond readily to medical or behavioral treatment, and so tend to be chronically institutionalized.

King refers to numerous studies of the neurological deficits in schizophrenia (and also autism) which link faulty vestibular and proprioceptive processing to schizophrenic symptoms. Some of these symptoms include perceptual deficits, feelings of fatigue and slow movement, postural insecurity (fear of falling), concrete thinking and lack of emotional response. King's hypothesis is that some schizophrenic patients have "defective proprioceptive feedback mechanisms, the vestibular component in particular being under-reactive in its role in the sensorimotor integration" (King 1974, 534).

Considering today's emphasis on the biochemical etiology of all mental illness (including schizophrenia), King's postulations of the circular role of movement in altering biochemical states as well as biochemistry affecting movement remains timely. Movement and sensation are known to produce chemical changes just as taking medication produces changes in brain chemistry. Furthermore, King states that "this model...applies not only to etiology but also to treatment. Although we cannot be sure which chemicals to alter, or in what direction, we can intervene in the motor behavior of the individual with the knowledge that there will be affects upon the thought processes and upon biochemistry" (King 1974, 534). In later publications, King notes the role of activities in coping with stress. A strenuous action, or "fight or flight" response to stress, (citing Gal and Lazarus 1975) was found to be responsible for the rapid metabolism of stress hormones, thus preventing secondary damage to the system. This suggests that strenuous or heavy work activity can serve to normalize the neurotransmitter balance which has been deranged by stress (King 1978, 1989).

The treatment techniques King utilizes in treating groups of chronic schizophrenic patients are adaptations of the techniques Ayres used with children. They are gross motor movement activities aimed at normalizing patterns of excessive flexion, adduction and internal rotation and increasing range of motion. Vestibular and tactile stimulation are provided through the use of the standard props - hammocks, scooter boards, balls and blankets. Heavy work patterns suggested by Rood (1974), resisted use of tonic muscle groups and cocontraction patterns are also incorporated. Other equipment King has added are parachutes, balloons and beanbag chairs.

King suggests two criteria for the selection of activities: 1) attention must not be centered upon the motor process, but rather on the object or outcome, and 2) the activity must be pleasurable, evoke smiles and laughter and a feeling of fun. Patients should not have to think about what they are doing or how they move; the goal is to elicit spontaneous movement and affect. Vestibular and proprioceptive processing occur at the brain stem level and produce automatic responses, not cortical (voluntary) responses. Therefore, if a ball is thrown to a patient and his hands extend spontaneously to catch it, we can assume that this automatic action reflects adaptive vestibular processing at the brain stem level. The goal of group activities using this frame of reference is to stimulate the sensory processing systems so that they will function more adaptively. As occupational therapists, we see spontaneous and purposeful motor responses as evidence that we are reaching that goal.

Ross

Mildred Ross further developed the use of sensory integrative theory and techniques with the chronic population. She extended the use of the sensory integration approach to the elderly, the neurologically impaired, the Alzheimer patient, the mentally retarded, and the long-term chronic patient of any age with disabilities that prevent adequate functioning in the community (Ross 1987). Ross developed her group techniques over more than 15 years of clinical experience. Her group sessions occur in five stages, which move developmentally from alerting activities involving tactile, kinesthetic and proprioceptive input to graded opportunities for organized cognitive thought and behavior. The following is a summary of Ross's five stage groups.

Stage I

Stage I acknowledges the presence of each member to each other member of the group. Introductions or saying names can easily accomplish this. The purpose of the session is established by the therapist or group members in stage I and this orients members to the session. Explanations should be kept brief, and on a level the members can understand. The attention of members should be captured in stage I.

Stage II

Stage II provides maximum exertion in movement. A variety of gross motor movement is suggested here, incorporating all three planes, horizontal, vertical and sagittal. Exercise, dance patterns or games may be adapted for this stage. Pleasure, communication and interaction or "cohesiveness" are possible goals. The effect of this stage is to stimulate or excite.

Stage III

Stage III emphasizes perceptual-motor skills. Activities may be chosen which require less vigorous movement and more judgment and focus action to accomplish a purposeful task. Making a fruit salad or drawing a picture are examples. The activities should be short-term and able to be finished in 30 minutes or less. This stage should have the effect of calming and focusing.

Stage IV

Stage IV is the time for cognitive stimulation. A discussion of the previous stages, memory games or poetry reading are suggested by Ross. "This is the opportunity for cortical controls to be demonstrated through organized behavior such as impulse control or creative expression. It is the highest point for display of attentiveness and group cohesiveness" (Ross 1987, 9). The length of this stage may be changed depending on the activity chosen and the level and interest of the group. Music or current events discussion may take a major portion of the time, while a short inspiring poem may take less than five minutes. Preparation for closure should be kept in mind in selecting activities for this stage.

Stage V

Stage V provides resolution and termination. A way to say goodbye, when to meet next or suggestions of what to do next time might serve as endings. When the therapist feels that the group was good, it may be appropriate to verbalize this in summarizing. Statements of satisfaction with the group by the therapist and patients can achieve a sense of peacefulness at its end.

Role of the Therapist

Using Ross's stages, the therapist plans and leads the activity, guided by knowledge of the principles of sensorimotor integration and activity analysis, but taking her cues from the group as well. The occupational therapist must be quite skilled to lead this kind of group effectively, keeping control while gently encouraging members to get involved. The stages provide a clear structure around which to plan appropriate activities. Ross, in her book, *Integrative Group Therapy* offers excellent guidelines for "considering when an activity should be introduced and how it should be presented" (Ross 1991).

Levy

Linda Levy (1974) provides another example of the use of the neurodevelopmental frame of reference. Levy uses Piaget's sensorimotor stage as her guide. Piaget asserts that in normal development, a child progresses through a series of stages which culminate in a mature understanding of reality (Piaget 1954). Adult psychotic patients, Levy states, mirror the characteristics of these stages. Mosey called this process the recapitulation of ontogeny, i.e., remission from psychosis is a replay of the original developmental process.

Several disorganized patients, Levy reports, have reverted to Piaget's earliest stage of learning, the sensorimotor stage (learning through movement). Four of the six stages that Piaget conceptualizes can serve as guidelines for occupational therapy groups (Figure 7-3). The following is a summary of Levy's four stage movement groups.

Stage 1 (birth-1 month)

In the beginning, the infant depends on reflex movement. Functional assimilation means the infant uses his available movements to perform a function, for example, sucking the breast. Generalizing assimilation occurs when the infant uses the same movement in new situations, i.e., sucking a bottle or pacifier.

Figure 7-3. Guidelines for movement activities. (Piaget's sensorimotor stages from Levy 1974.)

The occupational therapist can make contact with even the most regressed patient through movement. At Stage 1, using kinesthetic cues (touching and moving body parts), the therapist can use the patient's available schemata (rocking, for example), to begin to explore new situations (swaying, swinging). Almost any gross motor pattern displayed by the patient can be extended and generalized to new situations with the occupational therapist's guidance.

Stage 2 (1-4 months)

Here the infant is interested in new movement patterns and tends to repeat those movements that bring pleasurable responses. The occupational therapist can imitate the patient's movement patterns and help the patient establish a consistent sequence of movement, such as rocking, walking or running. This introduces a time sequence. Repetitive movement patterns can be applied to simplified sports, such as balloon volleyball, shuffleboard, basketball or games of catch. Movements that are habitual and reflexive in Stage 2 should be associated with a consistent result, e.g., the ball is caught and returned, the basketball goes through the hoop and bounces. The causal effect of movement is thus conveyed.

Stage 3 (4-10 months)

The infant looks for the effect of his actions on the external environment. For example, he may kick and discover that he makes his cradle rock. In stage 3, imitative exercise is appropriate, so the patient practices matching his movements to that of a model. Simple dance patterns and sequences are useful in groups at this stage, as long as they incorporate familiar movements. This stage is a precursor to the patient learning new skills through imitation.

Stage 4 (9-12 months)

The infant can imitate model behaviors. When mother pushes the teddy bear's stomach, it squeaks, so the infant tries it too. He imitates the action even if it doesn't have the same effect. When new learning becomes possible, the patient can apply his new skills to the more traditional task activities available in the occupational therapy clinic.

The sensorimotor stages described are thought to be necessary to precede mature cognition. The infant begins to elaborate on the basic dimensions of space, time and causality and relates them to movements. In this approach, Levy uses the development of the infant as a guide for planning motor activities that stimulate growth in the adult with mental illness who does not demonstrate normal cognitive functioning.

Function and Dysfunction

In the neurodevelopmental frame of reference, functioning is adequate when a person is able to learn and use all of the adaptive skills characteristic of his age. Since there is assumed to be a sequence of neurological and physiological development, dysfunction can be defined as a lag in development causing the patient to function below his age level. An adult is dysfunctional when neurological or physiological malfunctioning interferes with normal daily activity and a normal course of life development. This view of dysfunction in any illness encourages the identification of a physical cause. Even mental illness, as King and Levy have discussed, can respond to a neurodevelopmental treatment approach which follows the guidelines of early development. In using movement and games, the patient's active participation is encouraged to produce an adaptive response in activities that are purposeful.

Change and Motivation

Change in neurophysiological functioning is thought to be brought about through several methods. Physical activity can produce change through its effect on muscle tone, muscle strength and range of motion. Physical activity has also been shown to produce chemical changes; this is how the "runner's high" has been explained. During occupational therapy activities, change in brain and body function can be brought about through sensory stimulation and repetition of movement.

It must be remembered in this frame that change occurs in a specific sequence, and progresses stage by stage up the hierarchy toward maturity. In an illness which has left patients without normal movement patterns and sensory processing skills, a baseline level must be established through careful sensorimotor assessment. Then, through a repetition of the developmental sequence, sensory and motor components of activity can be utilized by the OT in such a way as to facilitate sub-cortical learning. Automatic movement and postural responses will precede more advanced cognitive responses. The changes we look for in the neurodevelopmental frame can often be seen as spontaneous self-corrections, such as an increased state of alertness or a more functional body posture. These normalized neurological states can then serve as building blocks for working on more skilled purposeful movements and the use of language in interactions within groups.

As Ross points out, activities we offer patients can have powerful effects on the central nervous system. These effects can be both positive and negative. Activities should be carefully planned to approach the central nervous system in a way that it can accept and handle, and to do so in a way that facilitates positive change. The occupational therapist does this through control and limitation of sensory input (Ross 1987).

Motivation comes in the form of accepting the challenge to be a more active participant in life. Patients, after illness or injury, may be motivated to go back to work, and to do things the way they used to. The lack of motivation comes when they expect too much change too fast, and therefore they feel they have failed. With long-term physical dysfunction, patients may be unable to modify their goals or accept new methods for meeting their needs. Chronic illness may leave patients without hope. When cognitive impairment accompanies the physical or emotional dysfunction, long-term goals may no longer be understood. The spontaneous urge to advance one's development must often be rekindled after illness. Interventions such as sensory stimulation and movement play can encourage the chronic patient to have more active participation with others and the environment. Once success or pleasure is experienced, patients may be more motivated.

Group Treatment

King, Ross and Levy, already cited, have given some helpful guidelines on how to structure groups. Gross motor activities are the common element. While movement activities are used extensively with pediatrics and physical dysfunction populations, movement is too often overlooked as an effective media for psychosocial dysfunction and geriatrics. As occupational therapists, we need to expand our repertoire of tools to include more activities involving movement. Much of our training in physiology, neuroanatomy and sensorimotor integration prepares us well for doing so. Perhaps our level of comfort in using movement with our patients is not as high as it could be. Often OTs need to be comfortable with their own ability to move and play before they are able to share this with patients.

Role of the Occupational Therapist

In the neurodevelopmental frame, the OT is a directive leader. The therapist needs a fairly thorough knowledge of neurodevelopment, neurophysiology and sensory integration in order to lead these groups competently. In most cases, patients we are working with are at low levels of functioning. Often verbal communication is at a minimum, and it is through imitation and role modeling that our patients perform activities therapeutically. The OT plans movement, sensory or cognitive activities that match their level and are relatively sure to succeed. The concept of the "just right challenge" applies here. Activities should interest and challenge the patients, but should not be so complex as to overwhelm them. In movement groups as described by King, Ross and Levy, the OT is the undeniable leader. She comes prepared with equipment and ideas and guides the group from start to finish, taking cues from patients as needed along the way.

Neurodevelopmentally based movement groups can be effective with some higher cognitive level populations as well. When this is done, care should be taken to explain the purpose thoroughly so that patients understand how the exercises and movements will help them.

Goals

Some of the goals mentioned by the various theorists may be summarized as follows.
1. Provide sensory stimulation and opportunities for adaptive response. The patient will develop skill in sensorimotor performance and strengthen normal sensorimotor integration.
2. Improve and maintain muscle tone, posture and motor planning. The patient will demonstrate these successfully during participation in activities.
3. Motivate the patient to participate. The patient will respond to stimulation by imitating or initiating activity.
4. Facilitate the development of higher level cognitive skills through the integration and assimilation of lower level skills. The patient will demonstrate higher level skills through participation in activity.
5. Achieve a sense of mastery and well-being. The patient will demonstrate positive affective responses during participation in activity.

Specific goals for individual patients may be easily set and measured. All of the goals may be worked on appropriately through the use of group activities.

Examples of Activities

Movement activities of all types may be adapted in this frame of reference, from simple calisthenics to dance and sports, to laying bricks and digging in the garden. When working with adult populations, the therapist must be careful not to make the activities seem too childish.

New Games

One particularly rich source of activities which are adaptable is the *Handbook of the New Games Foundation* (Fluegelman 1976). The New Games Foundation is an organization originating at San Francisco State College in 1966 as a resistance to the Vietnam War. The group was against any type of competition, even in sports. So they designed games which provided opportunities for individuals to express aggressiveness without anyone winning or losing. The games were designed for all ages and levels of activity, and since 1974, every few years they publish yet another book of newly invented games. Here are a few examples:

Blob

The Blob begins as a game of tag. When the person who is "it" catches someone, that person joins hands and becomes part of the Blob. Only the outside hand on either end of the Blob can snatch runaway players. Thus the insidious Blob keeps growing, cornering stray runners and forcing them to join up. In large groups, the Blob may split itself into parts and organize raiding parties to round up the last few strays. Boundaries must be set for this game, so eventually everyone is caught. "The thrilling climax occurs when there's only one player left to put up a heroic last ditch stand on behalf of humanity" (Fluegelman 1976, 107). The last survivor can start the next Blob as the game continues.

This game is obviously for people who are ambulatory, have good balance and coordination and have enough cognitive understanding to be able to follow simple rules. Blob is a simple concept that can be fun even for those who do not grasp its deeper implications. Done inside a room with the elderly, a therapist can talk the group through any difficulties, or he/she can begin by being the Blob. It may be done slowly or quickly to adapt to patient ability, and it provides light exercise with an element of fun and challenge.

People to People

Here is a new game which is made for occupational therapy. It is especially good for integrating movement, motor planning and cognition. Everyone chooses a partner and the game begins with a rhythmic clapping and snapping in unison (clap-clap-right hand snap-snap-left hand). The **caller** names two body parts, one on the right snap, the other on the left snap; for example, "elbow to ear." On the next snap-snap the whole group repeats "elbow to ear" while simultaneously one partner places his elbow on the other partner's ear. The caller continues to name body parts, trying to challenge the group by naming obscure anatomical structures (esophagus to gastrocnemius) or forcing them to take awkward positions. When the caller gets tired of this, he or she may call out "people to people." Then everyone must change partners, and in the confusion, the caller grabs a partner, leaving another member to become the new caller.

Adaptations for this game are endless. At the very least, it is a great socialization ice breaker, sure to get everyone laughing. It's also an excellent way for occupational therapy students to study their anatomy. Patients can practice bilateral coordination (clapping and snapping), motor planning (touching parts with partner), body awareness (identifying parts) and cognition (naming and recognizing body parts). A fair amount of balance, coordination and visual-motor integration are required to perform this activity successfully. Care should be taken with this and other games requiring touch that patients are not threatened by the close proximity to others.

The New Games followers suggest what occupational therapists already know. That all the games can be adapted by changing the rules, or that new games can be invented to meet the special needs and goals of our patients.

Parachute Games

King suggests parachute play as effective for spontaneous range of motion and postural correction as well as vestibular-proprioceptive stimulation (Figure 7-4). A real parachute (with no strings) works best and can be obtained in surplus stores or sports equipment supply catalogs.

All the games begin with group members holding an edge of the parachute at even intervals. It will take a few tries to move the parachute up over heads and down to the knees in unison to "catch the air." When the group has accomplished this, members can take turns running under the chute and exchanging places with one another across the circle. Other variations of parachute play are as follows:

Popcorn

When the parachute is down, a few tennis balls can be tossed in the center. The group makes the balls "pop" into the air and catches them with the parachute.

Round the World

One ball is placed in the center of the parachute. The group is instructed to work together to make the ball roll around the edge of the parachute by moving it in unison.

Down the Drain

Two colored balls are placed in the parachute. One side (blue ball) tries to get the other side's ball (red ball) to drop through the hole in the middle of the parachute.

Figure 7-4. Parachute play.

Secret Club

Billow the parachute by the unified above the head, below the knees motion of the group. Then on the count of three, group members bring the parachute edge down *behind* their backs and proceed to sit on the edge of the parachute. The air in the middle produces a "tent" in which the "secret club" can meet (but not for long or the air can get very stale!)

Shark

(This one is my favorite.) The members gather up the edge of the chute at just about waist level until a "calm sea" is produced. Then the "shark" ducks under and stalks the group with one finger pointing up touching the parachute from below, so that his movements may be observed from the top of the parachute. At an unexpected moment, the shark grabs the legs of an unsuspecting group member. The "victim" screams loudly as she is pulled under to become the next "shark." Two or three sharks at a time may be used in larger groups.

Parachute games are rich in sensory motor integration potential. The basic movement involved requires reaching high above the head, an extension of the shoulders, elbows and wrists to the full range of motion. The head tends to roll back as the patient looks at the effect of his movement, the parachute rising high in the air. Lowering the parachute to below the knee requires the patient to flex the spine forward at the waist and to extend the head forward, again following the movement of the parachute. The motion of the head and joints provides both proprioceptive and vestibular stimulation. Other movements may also be analyzed in this manner to aid in treatment planning to meet specific goals.

Bioenergetic Groups

These are groups aimed at the expression of feelings through movement. The major spokesman for this approach to movement is Alexander Lowen. Lowen's bioenergetic exercises were developed from his bioenergetic theory of personality, which is understood in terms of the body and it's energetic processes (Lowen 1977). More recently, Lowen's workshops have been offered as an extension of the myofacial release therapy workshops given by John Barnes, a physical therapist. Bioenergetic exercises can offer occupational therapists guidelines in the use of breathing and movement exercises to heighten emotional awareness and expression. Some of the bioenergetics exercises can release very powerful feelings, and should not be done without training. However, the basic concept is useful in planning expressive exercises in moderation. For further information about this approach, the reader is referred to Lowen's book *The Way to Vibrant Health* (1977).

The following activity groups are based on this concept, and have been used with adult psychiatric patients who are inhibited in the expression of feelings. In doing these activities, the occupational therapist should be careful not to overstimulate potentially volatile patients. The exercises should not be done with patients who are excitable or at risk for violent behavior. These neurophysiological techniques are especially well-suited to the treatment of depression.

Expressing Anger with Movement

Materials: exercise mats or thick carpeting, pillows.

Directions: Give directions for each step of the sequence and allow members to take the time they need for each step.

1. Lie down on your back on the mat and extend both legs. Kick your legs

rhythmically and allow your energy to flow into this motion. Take a few minutes to do this, setting your own pace.

2. Stand up and form a circle. Kick alternately with right, then left leg into the center of the circle.
3. Clench your fists and as you kick into the center of the circle, say "No!" Louder!
4. What other words can we say? As members make suggestions, have the whole group try them. Try punching into the center of the circle and saying words or making sounds.
5. Rest a few minutes and concentrate on breathing. Walk slowly around the circle, then turn and walk the other way. The slow walking has a calming effect after the excitement of kicking and punching.
6. Lie down on stomach with pillow in front of you. Punch pillow with right and left fists in a rhythmic motion. Do this for a few minutes and set your own pace.
7. As you punch the pillow, say "No!" If you feel like kicking also, allow yourself to do this.
8. If you would like, give the pillow a name. (Therapists should do this with caution, so as not to arouse too much anger).
9. After a few minutes wind down and just breathe slowly, resting head on pillow.
10. Stand up again when rested. Shrug shoulders in a backward roll and loosen tension in the neck area.
11. As patients shrug, say "Get off my back!" Louder!
12. Sit in a circle and massage muscles in back of neck. Each person massages the back of the person in front of him or her.

This exercise must be processed so that patients are not left with unresolved angry feelings. One goal is awareness of anger so that its appropriate expression can be discussed. Another goal is eliciting normal movement patterns subcortically. The careful planning and adaptation of this type of activity can utilize the concepts of Rood, NDT, PNF, Brunnstrom or sensory integration.

Acting Out Feelings

Materials: 20 index cards with feeling words, paper and pencils, stopwatch. Words for cards are: lonely, disgusted, excited, pleased, annoyed, infuriated, friendly, jealous, miserable, crabby, ecstatic, impatient, giddy, silly, moody, spacy, frightened, terrified, hopeless, hurt, anxious. Other feeling words may be added or substituted.

Directions: Each member draws a card and takes 30 seconds to act out the feeling on the card. Someone should be designated as timekeeper. Players may make sounds, but no words are allowed. Players can walk back and forth in front of the group, sit, stand, lie down, make gestures and facial expressions. The entire 30 seconds should be used. Non-verbal interaction with other members may be allowed as long as no one is hurt.

Members do not shout out their guesses; this is *not* charades. When time is up, group members write down what they think the feeling is. As each "mini-drama" ends, members read out their feeling words and discuss why they thought so. After a brief discussion, the player shows the group the card. Members continue to draw cards and act out feelings until they are all used.

Exercise Groups

Exercise to music or dance activities has good potential as a therapeutic tool. Circle or group dancing is usually best suited to our purpose in occupational therapy. In physical disability areas where goals involve maintaining and increasing strength and range of motion, group activities that accomplish these goals are more enjoyable and motivating than individual exercise programs. A good example of this type of group is the "Range of Motion Dance," an exercise program for patients with rheumatoid arthritis developed by Diane Harlowe and Patricia Yu at St. Mary's Hospital Medical Center in Madison, Wisconsin (Van Deusen & Harlowe, 1987). This is a guided fantasy done with groups of arthritis patients seated in chairs. The exercises, while following the story, go systematically through the range of motion for nearly every joint in the body. Once the sequence of motions is learned, it can be repeated by the patients at home by listening to the story on an audiotape. Greenfield and Godinez have introduced a similar group for stroke patients, called "self-range-of-motion (SROM) exercises" (Greenfield & Godinez, 1989). They have defined eight skill levels for these exercises, ranging from complete dependence on the therapist leader to independence in performing the exercises.

In doing such groups, it is important to use the potential of the group to provide mutual support, encouragement and feedback. Don't let the activity speak for itself; combine it with verbal reinforcement, progress checks and education about how and why it's helping. It is generally the social and emotional aspects of a group that keep members coming back.

Neurodevelopmental Therapy Groups with Handicapped Children

Sophie Levitt (1982) suggests therapeutic group work using a neruodevelopmental approach for children with cerebral palsy and motor delay. Both play groups and structured groups are seen as more effective than individual treatment for several reasons. The group often curtails rebellion and encourages cooperation. Children imitate other children and often instruct each other in doing what is required. Children seem to be able to concentrate longer with the stimulation of the group setting (one to one and a half hours as opposed to twenty minutes individually, Levitt reports), more than twice as long. Levitt emphasizes the interdisciplinary nature of these groups. Occupational and physical therapists, nurses, speech therapists and teachers all contribute to planning and implementing the activity.

In groups with handicapped children, it is not useful to group by diagnosis. Children should be selected for the groups according to their functional problems. The basis of selection may be motor problems such as poor grasp and release, poor balance or recurring abnormal movement patterns or postures. The developmental or cognitive level of group members should be similar. Some children who are too severely involved to be aware of the group may not be appropriate. The selected group should be capable of working together and establishing a degree of group spirit. The specific activities should be selected according to the deficits of the members (Levitt 1982).

It is evident that adults as well as children should be treated in groups of similar developmental level, and that the same principles for selection and planning apply. It would be encouraging to see more groups of physically disabled adults treated in a manner that encourages interaction and takes advantage of general group dynamics principles.

Music in Neurodevelopmental Groups

The use of music in therapy groups has been mentioned briefly. Music has qualities that can both relax and invigorate; it can energize a group, distract it or put it to sleep. The choice of music should be made with care, instrumental rather than vocal may be less distracting. The patients' level of stimulation should be closely monitored, as Ross suggests. Music can change the mood of the group, but the key is to do it gradually; the music should match the mood of the patients to begin with, and then change little by little, accompanied by appropriate movement activities. It can arouse emotion easily because it has an effect on the body and the mind. Selection of music may depend to a great extent on what you want to accomplish with the patient. With depressed patients, the therapist may want to energize them by playing music with a lively beat. Patients susceptible to anxiety might benefit more from slow mellow rhythms and ballads that soothe the nerves. In any case, occupational therapists usually use music in combination with movement activities, and it is the activity that should remain the focus with the music providing an appropriate background.

Group Leadership

Introduction

In neurodevelopmental groups, the explanation of purpose should match the patients ability to understand it. The level of cognition is the most important factor, and this varies widely in groups using the neurodevelopmental approach.

The warm-up is essential, and takes on a somewhat different emphasis here. The warm-up should prepare the members for the activity not only psychologically, but physiologically as well. As Ross has stressed, "there is a systematic way to approach the central nervous system"(1987). If members are unable to screen out non-essential sensory stimulation, they may be overloaded very quickly. With patient populations that are at risk for this, such as stroke and head trauma patients, autistic and developmentally delayed patients and the chronic mentally ill, the warm-up can offer limited and gradually increasing stimuli to test the group for an acceptable level of sensory stimulation.

Likewise, with the physically ill, the warm-up may be used as a testing experience to determine what level of physical exercise can be tolerated. Naturally the occupational therapist has evaluated the patient members prior to the group planning, so she should already be aware of the limits of safety. However, patients' conditions will vary on a daily (or hourly) basis and changes need to be taken into account. Based on the warm-up, the time frame or the activity itself may have to be modified.

Activity

The activities used will vary widely depending on the patient population. Sensorimotor or cognitive-perceptual tasks are most common. Activities will generally address some aspect of neurological or physical functioning and will facilitate some kind of adaptive response. Unlike previously described frames of reference, there may be several short-term activities planned during each session. The activities are organized and sequenced according to neurophysiological theory, so that simpler sensorimotor activities can build up to advanced, more complex activities. Likewise, high stimulation activities are followed by slower, more calming ones, so that the central nervous system does not get overstimulated. Timing depends on the endurance and attention span of members, and sessions can be relatively short, 30-50 minutes. Materials which facilitate movement, like mats, balls, props and pillows are often used. Craft activities or work activities which incorporate gross motor actions are also useful.

Sharing and Processing

Sharing in movement groups occurs within the bounds of the activity. Patients can observe each other's movements; the cognitive or symbolic meaning of the movement is really not the point, and therefore not necessary to share. Processing involves expressing feelings about the group, and when possible, should be done verbally. Verbal processing can reveal hidden resistances and bring out other problems patients have while participating in the activity, which are important to note.

Generalizing and Application

The principles learned are associated with the effects of activity or movement of various kinds on the body and the emotions. The knowledge of the therapist may be shared with the group, when appropriate, to facilitate this learning. For example, a group of depressed patients may notice that after the physical expression of anger and hostility, they feel more energy. The lesson in this is that expression of feeling is natural and healthy. The application is to find ways to express feeling without hurting others or otherwise getting into trouble.

Application, even with lower functioning patients, may involve learning to repeat a desired adaptive response. When movement activities result in spontaneous laughter, for example, the pleasure of this response may motivate the patient to repeat the movement that produced it. The neurodevelopmental response to movement activities tends to be spontaneous, and not planned. As patients integrate new movement patterns into their repertoire, they will use them spontaneously at times outside of the group. The goal is to stimulate the development of higher level skills, and more adaptive functioning in the patient's everyday life.

Neither generalization nor application need to be separate phases of the neurodevelopmental group. The verbal summary is sufficient to reinforce this learning.

Bibliography

Ayres AJ. *The Development of Sensory Integrative Theory and Practice*. Dubuque, IA: Kendall Hunt, 1974.

Bobath B. The neurodevelopmental approach to treatment, in Pearson P. (ed.) *Physical Therapy Services in Developmental Disabilities*. Springfield, IL: Charles Thomas, 1972.

Brunnstrom, S. *Movement Therapy in Hemiplegia*. New York: Harper & Row, 1970.

Eggers, O. *Occupational Therapy in the Treatment of Adult Hemiplegia*. London: William Heinemann Medical Books, 1983.

Fisher A. and Bundy A. *Sensory Integration*. Philadelphia, FA Davis, 1991.

Fluegelman A. New games foundation. *The New Games Book*. Garden City, NY: Doubleday, 1976.

Gal R. and Lazarus RS. The role of activity in anticipating and confronting stressful situations. *J of Human Stress* 1975, 4, 4-20.

Greenfield JM. and Godinez M. Stroke clients learn independence by leading their own therapy group. *OT Week* (AOTA) April 20, 1989.

King LJ. A Sensory-Integrative Approach to Schizophrenia, *AJOT* 1974, 28, 9, 529-536.

King LJ. Toward a Science of Adaptive Responses, Slagle Lecture, *AJOT* 1978, 32, 7, 9-437.

King LJ. Occupational therapy and neuropsychiatry in *Mental Health Focus*, Rockville, MD. AOTA, 1988.

Levitt S. *Treatment of Cerebral Palsy and Motor Delay*, Boston: Blackwell Scientific Publications, 1982

Levy LL. Movement Therapy for Psychiatric Patients *AJOT* 1974, 28, 6, 354-357.

Lowen A. and Lowen L. *The Way to Vibrant Health*, New York: Harper and Row, 1977.

Lloens L. Theoretical Conceptualizations of Occupational Therapy: 1960-1982 *OT in Mental Health*, 1984, (2)1-14.

Ross M. *Group Process: Using Therapeutic Activities in Chronic Care*, Thorofare NJ: SLACK Inc., 1987.

Trombly C. *Occupational Therapy for Physical Dysfunction*. 3rd ed. Baltimore: Williams and Wilkins, 1989.

Van Deusen J. and Harlowe D. The Efficacy of the ROM Dance Program for Adults with Rheumatoid Arthritis *AJOT* 1987, 41, 2, 90-95.

Chapter

8

A Model of Human Occupation Approach

The model of human occupation (MOHO) emerged around 1980 as a further definition of the theory of occupational behavior developed by Mary Reilly (1962). The central idea of occupational behavior theory is that engagement in activity or occupation in itself will produce and maintain health. Human achievement and daily occupation are identified as the focal point for the development of the model of human occupation (Kielhofner 1988). White (1959) is credited with introducing the concept of the human need for competence and achievement. Kielhofner, Burke and Igi (1980) expanded on these concepts and combined them with general systems theory. They describe the human being as an open system, define the various parts of the system (volitional, habituation and performance subsystems) and describe how it interacts with other systems (culture, tasks, social norms, human and non-human environment). The MOHO can be viewed as a superstructure which organizes concepts and expresses them in terms which can be readily applied to assessment and treatment.

Basic Assumptions

The Human Open System

The basic assumption in applying systems theory to human functioning is that man is an open system that can change and develop through interaction with the environment. The human open system is described as a cyclical process involving output, feedback, input and throughput (Kielhofner & Burke, 1985). The human being gives output to the environment, receives feedback in the form of input from the environment and experiences throughput, a process of change and adaptation of the person resulting from the feedback given. The system is divided into parts for the purpose of examining (assessment) and influencing (treatment) its processes.

The Three Subsystems

Following systems theory, throughput occurs within the structures of three hierarchical subsystems. The **volitional** subsystem controls the overall operations of the system in choosing and initiating occupational behavior. The **habituation** subsystem organizes occupational behavior into role patterns and routines. The lowest subsystem is **performance**, the production level of behavior, providing skills and motor capacities to carry out occupational behavior. The three sub-systems work together in an integrated fashion to maintain the balance of work, play and self-care activities.

The Volitional Subsystem

At the top of the hierarchy, this system serves a control function in energizing the other subsystems toward desired goals. The three main components of this subsystem are personal causation, values and interests. **Personal causation** refers to a belief in oneself, and is related to feelings of competence. A healthy individual is thought to possess needed skills, and to believe him or herself to be capable of using these skills to have a desired effect on the environment. A person who believes in him or herself expects to succeed through the use of his or her own abilities. A person who lacks a sense of personal causation may feel that what happens is controlled by fate or external circumstance. Such a person feels helpless to cope with the functional problems resulting from illness and disability.

Values in the model of human occupation refer to the meaningfulness of activities. Individuals are thought to spend time doing activities that have meaning, and are thought to be good or morally right. For example, if a student thinks that having a college degree is good, he may work very hard at reading, writing and studying, activities that will help him achieve that goal. Patients often find themselves unable to perform activities that they consider to be important or meaningful, such as going back to work. A re-prioritizing of values might be a treatment goal. Using this model, patients can find alternate ways to perform a work role that are within their capabilities.

Interests in this model are defined as tendencies to find certain occupations pleasurable. If a person enjoys a particular activity, he may be inclined to participate in it frequently, or for longer periods of time. Interests relate to work, play and self-care activities, and are not limited to recreational endeavors. A healthy individual uses his interests to guide present action, and to plan his use of time. A person lacking in interests may need help in exploring his environment and in finding pleasure in activities.

In summary, the volitional subsystem guides the occupational behavior of the individual in ways that are meaningful and pleasurable, and are likely to have a desired effect on the environment.

The Habituation Subsystem

The concept of habit training dates back to the writings of Adolph Meyer (1922). He describes the "systematic engagement of interest and concern about the actual use of time and work (as) an obligation and a necessity" in the treatment of chronic illness (Meyer, 1922, *AJOT* 1977, 640). The organization of activities throughout the day is the concern of the habituation subsystem, as conceptualized by the MOHO. Roles and habits are its components.

A **role** is a position or status within a social group, along with its accompanying obligations and expectations. Some typical roles are worker, parent, family member, student and volunteer. Functional individuals generally play a variety of life roles, and find it necessary to achieve a balance of these if they are to maintain order in their lives. The roles we play have an organizing effect on how we use time. The worker role and the family member role, for example, each require the performance of defined tasks which must be balanced and planned for if the day is to flow smoothly. Our patients may lack social roles, or may find it difficult to meet the obligations and expectations of their roles. The focus of therapy may be the development of new roles and/or the planning and modification of activities required within chosen roles.

Habits are routine or typical ways in which a person performs tasks. For example, a morning routine may involve getting up at 7am, bathing, dressing and eating breakfast. Habits can decrease the effort required to perform tasks by making them so routine that they are almost automatic. Consider the effort needed to find one's way to a new place of work. After driving the same route for several days, one recognizes familiar landmarks and the trip requires much less conscious thought. This routine allows the individual to save his energy for the more challenging activities of the day. Illness often results in a breakdown of normal routines. Occupational therapy may be needed to re-learn and reorganize one's habits after illness.

The Performance Subsystem

This subsystem includes all of the skills required to perform purposeful activities. Three types of skills are identified: perceptual-motor, process and communication/interaction skills. A person's performance is directly linked to the output of the human open system. Although the performance subsystem is the lowest level in the hierarchy, the higher levels can only perform to the extent that existing skills will allow. Therefore, a lack of skills can prevent the needed organization of roles and habits, the pursuit of interests and the accomplishment of valued goals.

Interaction With the Environment

The three subsystems discussed above are part of the throughput process of the human open system. Output, feedback and input define the system's interaction with the environment. Since the health and adaptation of the individual is dependent on this interaction, the environment represents a vital part of the model of human occupation. The model defines the components of the environment as objects, tasks, social groups and organizations and culture. These are sometimes referred to as environmental layers, because they represent progressively wider and more abstract levels of environmental awareness.

Environmental **press** is the expectation of performance or behavior placed on an individual by a given environment (Baris, 1985). For example, a health club environment requires the individual to dress in a defined manner, and to demonstrate a certain level of physical skill. Individuals generally seek out environments which fit their interests and their level of skill. Individuals who are disabled may find themselves in environments which do not match their competence level, and may need the services of an occupational therapist to help them change either their skill level or their environment.

A general outline for organizing data about the human open system is found in Table 8-1.

For definitions and elaboration of all these terms the reader is referred to Kielhofner's, *A Model of Human Occupation*. Proponents of the MOHO as a frame of reference

---

Table 8-1.
Components of the Model of Human Occupation

I. Volitional Subsystem
  A. Personal causation
    1) belief in skill
    2) belief in efficacy of skill
    3) expectancy of success/failure
    4) internal/external control
  B. Values
    1) temporal orientation
    2) meaningfulness of activity
    3) occupational goals
    4) personal standards
  C. Interests
    1) discrimination
    2) pattern
    3) potency
II. Habituation Subsystem
  A. Roles
    1) perceived incumbancy
    2) internalized expectations
    3) balance

  B. Habits
    1) degree of organization
    2) social appropriateness
    3) flexibility/rigidity
III. Performance Subsystem
  A. Skills
    1) interpersonal/communication
    2) process (planning-problem solving)
    3) perceptual motor
  B. Skill constituents
    1) symbolic
    2) neurological
    3) musculoskeletal
IV. The Environment
  A. Physical space/objects
  B. Persons
  C. Tasks
  D. Cultural and social norms

Adapted with permission from Kielhofner, *A Model of Human Occupation.* Baltimore, Williams and Wilkins 1985.

claim that the above outline can be applied to any age group or disability area treated in occupational therapy. Other frames of reference may be used within its context, such as sensory integration (Mack, Lindquist and Parham 1982). Motivation in this frame of reference is attributed to an innate urge to explore and master the environment. Many writers have been credited with the elaboration of this concept, which is said to have a biological basis (Kielhofner 1989). The best known of these is R.H. White (1960) who contributed the ideas of competence, adaptation and motivation.

Levels of Occupational Functioning

The model specifies three levels of occupational functioning: exploration, competence and achievement (Reilly 1974). These have also been called levels of arousal and accomplishment (Kielhofner 1988, Kaplan 1986). Exploration is the lowest level, and involves curious investigation of oneself and one's potential for action in conjunction with the properties of the environment. Competence involves striving to meet the demands of a situation through the development of skills and their organization. Achievement includes striving for excellence and the successful performance of roles.

Concurrent levels of occupational dysfunction are also described as inefficacy, incompetence and helplessness. Inefficacy, the least dysfunctional level, implies a reduction of motivation.

Function and Dysfunction

When the human open system is functioning optimally, order exists within the system. This means that the individual competently performs everyday tasks of daily life in a routine and satisfying way (Rogers 1982). This "order" produces and maintains a state of health in the individual. If a person can describe a typical day at work or home, identify a number of social roles he performs and express satisfaction with these, then he is seen to be healthy.

Disorder is the opposite; it's a lack of order in one's life which can be seen in dysfunctional daily routines, a lack of social roles and/or dissatisfaction with any aspect of the person's life structure. When disorder exists, the occupational therapist evaluates the patient to determine what parts of the system are not operating properly. Barris, Kielhofner and Watts (1983) suggest several specific kinds of disorder, including open system dysfunction, disruption in intrinsic motivation, poor decision-making capacity, role dysfunction, temporal dysfunction, disorder of environmental interactions and disorder of performance components.

There are dozens of assessment tools originating from this frame of reference, which can help OTs to specify which parts of the system are disordered or malfunctioning. The state of order or disorder is easily observed in the patient's occupational behavior.

Change and Motivation

Change in the MOHO involves the restoration of order in the person's internal and external life structure. In recovering from illness, this often means restructuring a person's daily routines and re-establishing role performance. For example, Angie's roles were secretary, wife and mother of a five-year-old son. When at age 35 she was hospitalized for depression following a bitter divorce, all of her roles became inactive. The occupational therapist collaborated with Angie in restructuring her life so that she could resume her roles as worker and mother. Angie was able to volunteer while in the hospital to help maintain her secretarial skills. She arranged to have dinner with her son each evening and to take him on an outing one day on the weekend. In restoring these roles, Angie was able to organize her already existing skills into a normal daily routine. She showered and dressed each morning, went to her volunteer job each day and met her son at a relative's house for dinner each evening. At night, she returned to the hospital.

The preceding therapy program addressed the components of the habituation and performance subsystems. Grieving over the loss of her role as spouse was dealt with in counseling and resulted in the addition of several activities to allow Angie to make new social contacts, like joining a tennis club and playing three times a week, and attending weekly meetings of a church social club.

The therapeutic work is not what activity is chosen, but in getting Angie moving toward the regular performance of desired occupational behaviors. Normal, everyday activities are the media used, and the patient herself makes the choices of activity, with the help and guidance of the occupational therapist.

My own opinion is that the major value of the MOHO lies in its holistic view of the individual and its helpfulness in organizing data about patients' specific dysfunctions. Many examples exist in the literature of the application of the MOHO in identifying patterns of occupational dysfunction.

Group Treatment

Most of the literature on the MOHO does not address group treatment specifically. However, several aspects of its superstructure are helpful in program planning. A balanced occupational therapy program is assured, for example, when one incorporates group activities addressing the areas of self-care, work and leisure. Another concept was to organize a program by using the three levels of occupational functioning. Kathy Kaplan (1986) writes about a group program for short-term psychiatry using group activities at the levels of exploration, competence and achievement.

Exploration level groups incorporate simple activities to help the most severely disorganized patients to develop basic process skills (planning and problem solving), perceptual motor skills and communication/interaction skills. The occupational therapist selects the activities and organizes the environment. The group is structured in four stages: 1) orientation and introductions 2) warm-up activities 3) selected activities 4) wrap-up. Kaplan calls this type of group a "directive group." An exercise group is another example of an explorative level group.

At the competence level, it is assumed that the patients have basic skills but may need to integrate them into habit patterns: "These groups are designed to help patients identify goals, interests and needs for meaning and action" (Kaplan 1986, 476). Some examples of groups at this level are task groups and activity planning groups.

Groups at the achievement level are designed to help patients integrate skills into daily life roles (Kaplan 1986). Examples of achievement level groups are assertiveness training and leisure awareness. For more information on the directive group the reader is also referred to Kaplan's *Directive Group Therapy* (1988).

The components of the three subsystems also suggest many possibilities for group treatment.

Group Structure and Limitations

It has been shown that the use of the MOHO is not limited by age or diagnosis. Functional levels are organized by levels of arousal and achievement and by the components of the three subsystems that are functioning within the human open system. The MOHO offers little in the way of group structure. It may be assumed that patients should be grouped homogeneously, according to their level of organization and specific deficit areas. The focus of occupational therapy in the MOHO is on activities and tasks and not on emotions or process.

Role of the Therapist

The therapist in the model of human occupation plays the role of an adviser and collaborator. She counsels the patients in the various aspects of occupational functioning. Kaplan's "directive group" is so named because of the "active and supportive way in which the group leaders elicit adaptive behaviors and structure the environment to assure maximum participation of all the members" (Kaplan 1986, 477). This role of leader as "director" is necessary for groups that have severely disorganized occupational behavior. However, even at this level, the occupational therapist encourages the active participation of the patients. The OT continues at higher levels to facilitate, not direct. Thus, the patients' sense of control and personal efficacy is reinforced by the occupational therapist as he/she continues to acquire new skills and make personal choices.

Goals

Goals are not discussed as a separate issue in the model of human occupation. Treatment goals are concerned with performance of normal daily occupations: work, daily living tasks and play. They may involve any or all of the three subsystems. In the volitional subsystem, exploration of values and rekindling the urge to explore and master the environment may be goals. Habit formation or the acquisition of new roles may be goals in the habituation subsystem. Learning and practicing the skills necessary to perform the tasks of one's chosen or valued roles can be goals in the performance subsystem.

Examples of Activities

The model of human occupation stresses the use of the patient's normal daily activities as the modalities of choice. Specialized equipment and techniques are not considered necessary, although they may be utilized to address special problems. The more common media used in therapeutic groups include cooking, money management, home maintenance skills, leisure planning and work skills. The patient's own interests guide activity selection and the focus is on the real problems of everyday living. Some kinds of activities necessitate longer sessions. The environment is important in providing feedback to the patient and challenging him to further exploration.

Some activities used in a program based on the model of human occupation are described here.

The Special Events Group

This group is designed for exploratory level patients (chronic mentally ill) whose social relations and daily routines are severely disordered. The purpose is to increase orientation, to expand their level of awareness to the world outside themselves, and to work on time planning and social skills. The focus is on events in peoples' lives, such as holidays, birthdays, welcomings and goodbyes, and how to celebrate them. The group is organized by the month, and begins with a planning session at the beginning of each month. The group meets for two hour sessions.

Materials and equipment: Poster board with lines drawn up like a monthly calendar. Other materials are colored markers, colored paper, scissors, glue, blank cards and envelopes, cake mixes and frosting ingredients, large sheet cake pan, cake decorating kit, two large punch bowls, ingredients for punch, cake knife, serving ladle, paper supplies for parties, birthday candles, coffee maker, cream and sugar and access to a kitchen for baking.

Directions: (for a typical month, October)

Week 1: Organize monthly calendar (Figure 8-1.)
- Write name of month and numbers. Therapist begins by writing #1 on the day the month begins.
- Identify season; decorate calendar with designs appropriate for the season: pumpkins, cornstalks, leaves.
- Identify holidays for that month, write on calendar or decorate with appropriate symbols.
- Survey all patients and staff on ward to find out whose birthday is in October, write on calendar.
- Identify one day for the whole ward to celebrate October birthdays and Halloween, write on calendar.

October						
S	**M**	**T**	**W**	**Th**	**F**	**S**

Figure 8-1. Special events group monthly calendar.

- Post the calendar in a prominent place on the ward. Other events such as discharge dates, arrival or departure of staff, may also be added.
- Plan what tasks need to be done for the celebration and decide when to do each. For example, make cards, bake cake, shop for supplies, think about masks or costumes for Halloween theme.

Week 2: Make cards
- Identify birthday people and write names on index cards.
- Each member makes one card. If there are not enough birthdays, make some for Halloween too. Each patient designs the card and writes the name and message inside. Stencils and markers, colored paper shapes, scissors and glue should be available for the less "artistic."
- Patients then circulate around the ward gathering signatures for the cards.
- A shopping list is made for needed refreshment items, eggs and milk for cake, ingredients for punch, etc. (The therapist does the actual shopping.)

Week 3: Bake cake and decorate
- Group meets in kitchen. Needed items should be set out on table ahead of time, bowls, mixing spoons, measuring cups and spoons, eggs, confectionery sugar, cake decorating supplies, etc. The large sheet cake pan holds two complete cake mixes, so the recipe should be doubled (assuming a ward size of twenty or more).
- The group divides into work teams and roles to accomplish this.
- Cake bakers: recipe reader, measurer, mixer, timer
- Frosting makers: recipe reader, measurer, mixer
- Designers: choose motif or theme, border design, colors and message.
- Supply frosting makers with desired food colors, trace motif design on paper (jack-o'lantern) and cut out. Write out message on paper and check spelling "Happy Birthday" and "Happy Halloween."(Figure 8-2.)
- Members learn to use decorating kit to decorate cake, frost in white, do border, trace motif and write message. All may help with this "fun" part, and all help clean up.
- When finished, the entire cake is frozen to be used the next week.
- The ward is informed of the date and the exact time and place are decided at a ward community meeting. Permission of staff is necessary.

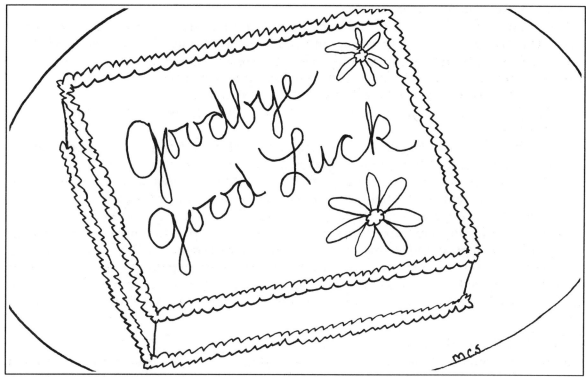

Figure 8-2. Cake decoration.

Week 4: Celebration

Preparation, one hour
- Take cake out of freezer two hours ahead.
- Cover a large table with a sheet in the party room.
- Set up chairs in a large circle.
- Set out punch bowls, make punch.
- Make coffee in coffee maker, set out cream and sugar.
- Set out plates, forks, cake knife, cake, cups, ladle, spoons and napkins.
- Bring the cards. Put the birthday candles on the cake. Bring matches or a lighter.

When everything is ready, gather patients and staff.

Party, 30 minutes
- Give a toast. Members serve everyone punch, but don't drink it right away, save it for the toast.
- The whole group is asked to take turns proposing toasts or sharing wishes with honored members.
- Members lead group in singing "Happy Birthday".
- Candles are lit.
- Birthday people must come forward and blow out candles.
- Group members serve cake to all. Members serve themselves last.

Informal socializing occurs while cake is being served. People help themselves to more punch or coffee. Clean up, discussion, 30 minutes.

All members help clean up. When finished, group gathers in a meeting room to discuss/evaluate: review what roles members played, give feedback, verbalize what skills were learned, discuss how to apply skills.

Vocational Readiness Group

This group uses craft or office activities to explore interests and practice work-related skills. The group runs for four weeks and has been used with competence level acute psychiatric patients and substance abuse patients. Appropriate members are those whose goal is to take on a work role after discharge. Group meets in two hour sessions.

The goals of the group involve all three MOHO subsystems.

a. Volitional: patients identify and explore their interests by selecting to do craft or office tasks.

b. Habituation: patients gain and/or maintain good work habits, such as punctuality and following directions, in anticipation of regaining the worker role.

c. Performance: patients practice basic work skills such as concentration, organization of time and materials, quality of workmanship and task follow-through. Specific skills like typing and woodworking may also be learned and practiced.

Materials and equipment: two typewriters, access to a copy machine, file cabinet with files and labels, typing tutorial manual, typing paper, workbench with vise, electric drill, band saw, pine boards, plywood, wood patterns, sandpaper, painting supplies, leather work supplies, belt blanks and key fob blanks, buckles, rivets, stamping tools, punch, mallets, bowls of water, sponges, written directions for making several projects at several different levels of complexity.

Week 1: Evaluation and Project Choice

Members begin by doing an activity checklist (Figure 8-3). The basis for this is Noomi Katz's adaptation of Matsutsuyu's Interest Checklist (1969), (Katz 1988.) For this group, the checklist has been modified to include work-related activities. The scale has been designed to include five work categories as follows:

1. Office work	2. Building and construction	3. Communication/teaching
typing	electrical wiring	writing articles
using computers	pipe fitting	making posters
filing	assembling parts	painting signs
answering phones	working on cars	broadcasting news
using calculator	house painting	introducing people
accounting & math	woodworking	reading books
writing letters	refinishing furniture	giving lectures
opening mail	installing carpeting	giving exams
making appointments	landscaping	taking notes
supervising employees	gardening	teaching children

4. Sales/service	5. Home maintenance
writing articles	showing houses
washing dishes	selling clothing
mopping floors	doing make-up
cooking	serving food
wallpapering	styling hair
arranging furniture	giving sales pitch
grocery shopping	giving fashion shows
menu planning	travel planning
doing laundry	dining with clients
mixing drinks	planning conferences
washing windows	

Activity	Interest			Past Performance			Future	
	some	casual	none	usual	some	never	yes	no
typing	☐	☐	☐	☐	☐	☐	☐	☐
electrical wiring	☐	☐	☐	☐	☐	☐	☐	☐
writing articles	☐	☐	☐	☐	☐	☐	☐	☐
showing houses	☐	☐	☐	☐	☐	☐	☐	☐
washing dishes	☐	☐	☐	☐	☐	☐	☐	☐
using computers	☐	☐	☐	☐	☐	☐	☐	☐
pipe fitting	☐	☐	☐	☐	☐	☐	☐	☐
making posters	☐	☐	☐	☐	☐	☐	☐	☐
selling clothing	☐	☐	☐	☐	☐	☐	☐	☐
mopping floors	☐	☐	☐	☐	☐	☐	☐	☐
filing	☐	☐	☐	☐	☐	☐	☐	☐
assembling parts	☐	☐	☐	☐	☐	☐	☐	☐
painting signs	☐	☐	☐	☐	☐	☐	☐	☐
doing make-up	☐	☐	☐	☐	☐	☐	☐	☐
cooking	☐	☐	☐	☐	☐	☐	☐	☐
answering phones	☐	☐	☐	☐	☐	☐	☐	☐
working on cars	☐	☐	☐	☐	☐	☐	☐	☐
news broadcasting	☐	☐	☐	☐	☐	☐	☐	☐
serving food	☐	☐	☐	☐	☐	☐	☐	☐
wallpapering	☐	☐	☐	☐	☐	☐	☐	☐
using calculator	☐	☐	☐	☐	☐	☐	☐	☐
woodworking	☐	☐	☐	☐	☐	☐	☐	☐
introducing people	☐	☐	☐	☐	☐	☐	☐	☐
styling hair	☐	☐	☐	☐	☐	☐	☐	☐
arranging furniture	☐	☐	☐	☐	☐	☐	☐	☐
accounting and math	☐	☐	☐	☐	☐	☐	☐	☐
refinishing furniture	☐	☐	☐	☐	☐	☐	☐	☐
reading books	☐	☐	☐	☐	☐	☐	☐	☐
giving sales pitch	☐	☐	☐	☐	☐	☐	☐	☐
menu planning	☐	☐	☐	☐	☐	☐	☐	☐
writing letters	☐	☐	☐	☐	☐	☐	☐	☐
installing carpeting	☐	☐	☐	☐	☐	☐	☐	☐
giving lectures	☐	☐	☐	☐	☐	☐	☐	☐
giving fashion shows	☐	☐	☐	☐	☐	☐	☐	☐
doing laundry	☐	☐	☐	☐	☐	☐	☐	☐
opening mail	☐	☐	☐	☐	☐	☐	☐	☐
landscaping	☐	☐	☐	☐	☐	☐	☐	☐
giving exams	☐	☐	☐	☐	☐	☐	☐	☐
travel planning	☐	☐	☐	☐	☐	☐	☐	☐
mixing drinks	☐	☐	☐	☐	☐	☐	☐	☐
making appointments	☐	☐	☐	☐	☐	☐	☐	☐
gardening	☐	☐	☐	☐	☐	☐	☐	☐
taking notes	☐	☐	☐	☐	☐	☐	☐	☐
dining with clients	☐	☐	☐	☐	☐	☐	☐	☐
supervising employees	☐	☐	☐	☐	☐	☐	☐	☐
teaching children	☐	☐	☐	☐	☐	☐	☐	☐
planning conferences	☐	☐	☐	☐	☐	☐	☐	☐
washing windows	☐	☐	☐	☐	☐	☐	☐	☐

Figure 8-3. Work activity checklist.

The checklist is discussed with regard to interests, past work history and satisfaction with current work skills. The expectations for the group are then shared (Figure 8-4.). Members are expected to:

    arrive on time or give prior notification of absence;
    appear well-groomed and dressed in clean work clothes;
    follow directions for project/task;
    respond positively to supervision;
    effectively deal with frustration;
    ask for help when needed;
    work independently;
    learn necessary skills;
    follow through on task (meet deadlines);
    strive for quality of workmanship.

Several starter projects should be ready with written directions for each patient. Members may choose projects based on their interests and skills, and get started for the remaining time. Examples of starter craft projects are leather key fobs with stamped initials and border, wood wall plaque made from pre-cut 6"x 8" pine board with picture to decoupage, or a wood trivet made from a kit. Examples of starter work projects are typing a short letter or sorting tiles by color. Starter projects are intended to teach basic skills and allow the therapist to evaluate patients' manual and cognitive ability.

Weeks 2, 3 and 4

Patients complete projects as assigned by the therapist. Each patient works independently on a different project. At the end of each session, members are evaluated with the Work Behavior Rating Scale (Figure 8-4), and results are discussed with the patients.

Group Leadership

In this frame of reference the activity or occupation itself is considered health-producing, and the need to take great pains to share it or understand its process is de-emphasized. In keeping with the greater emphasis on activities, two steps in the seven step process have been eliminated: sharing and processing. There are longer and more frequent group meetings and activities tend to be longer or ongoing, so that discussions of general principles and application are not necessary during every session. However, the introduction and summary should be done without fail, and should serve the purposes outlined in Chapter 1.

Introduction

Greetings and description of the purpose are done thoroughly at the outset of each activity. A warm-up is optional and can be used to set the mood or energize patients if appropriate. The expectations may be general and somewhat tentative as the members will have input and make choices as the group progresses. The time frame often varies according to the activity and therefore should be started at the beginning of each session.

	Dates				
Name:					
Arrives on time (gives prior notice of valid absence)					
Appropriate appearance (well-groomed, clean work clothing)					
Follows directions					
Responds positively to supervision					
Effectively deals with frustration					
Asks for help when needed					
Works independently					
Learns necessary skills					
Follows through on tasks (meets deadlines)					

Scale: 1=independent and correct
2=requires some assistance
3=requires much assistance
4=is dependent or unmotivated

Figure 8-4. Work behavior rating scale.

Activity

At the exploratory level, the activities selected for groups are generally designed to help patients develop specific skills. Patients who need to work on these skills are grouped together. For example, those who need to develop routines for self-care might do a series of skill building sessions such as maintaining finger and toe nails, doing laundry, selecting appropriate clothing, applying make-up/shaving, care of teeth, care of hair and skin.

At the competence level, choices are encouraged so that patients can apply their skills and organize them into habit patterns (Kaplan 1986). Patients may be encouraged to set their own goals within the group context. For example, the title of the group may be "time management," and within that theme, patients may plan their own individual time schedules.

Achievement level groups focus on life roles such as: work support, leisure planning and values clarification.

Generalizing and Application

The meaning of the activity is discussed with the group as outlined in Chapter 1. This is done after the activity is completed, and focuses on how the activity relates to the life roles of the members. Similarities and differences among group members is de-emphasized. For example, in the vocational readiness group described earlier, the skills learned in doing a leather craft project may be generalized to a patient's actual job. Concentration, efficient use of tools, work neatness and finishing on time are skills necessary for both. This kind of discussion leads directly into application. A group discussion in the vocational readiness group will necessarily focus on individual application of skills, as patients' vocational plans differ widely. Feedback from the occupational therapist from the vocational rating scale should also be presented in the group. The group focus is useful to confirm the therapist's observations and give a stronger message to patients. For example, a member may have done very careful work, and showed considerable manual skills, but he may have taken excessive time to do so. The reality of the workplace is not only to do quality work, but also to meet deadlines. The group discussion may help the patient see the necessity to compromise and perhaps curb his perfectionistic tendencies.

Summary

The summary should review the purpose and goals of the group, and determine what the group accomplished. Focus on individual achievements and strengths should be confirmed. The skills learned may be general or different for each member, and their application should be reinforced in the summary. Future plans, goal achievement and life roles to which occupational therapy activities apply may be discussed by each member as part of the summary.

Bibliography

Barris R, Kielhofner G & Watts J *Psychosocial Occupational Therapy: Practice in a Pluralistic Arena*, Laurel, Md., Ramsco, 1983.

Bruce MA & Borg B *Frames of Reference in Psychosocial Occupational Therapy*, Thorofare NJ: SLACK Inc., 1987.

Kaplan K The Directive Group: Short-term Treatment for Psychiatric Patients with a Minimal Level of Functioning, *AJOT* 1986, 40,7,474-481

Kaplan K *Directive Group Therapy*, Thorofare, NJ: SLACK Inc., 1988.

Katz N. Interest Checklist: A Factor Analytical Study, *O.T. in Mental Health*, 1988, 1, 45-55.

Kielhofner G. General Systems Theory: Implications for Theory and Action in Occupational Therapy, *AJOT*, 1988, 32,10,637-645.

Kielhofner G, Burke J. & Igi C. A Model of Human Occupation, part 4. *AJOT*, 1980, 34,12,572-581.

Kielhofner G., Ed.*A Model of Human Occupation: Theory and Application*. Baltimore: Williams and Wilkins, 1985.

Kielhofner G. Model of Human Occupation, in Robinson S, Ed., *Mental Health Focus*, Rockville, MD: AOTA, 1988.

Lindquist J., Mack W. & Parham L.D. A synthesis of occupational behavior and Sensory Integration Concepts in Theory and Practice, Part 2: Clinical applications. *AJOT*. 1982, 36,7,433-437.

Mack W., Lindquist J. & Parham L.D. A Synthesis of occupational behavior and sensory integration concepts in theory and practice, Part 1: Theoretical foundations. *AJOT*, 1982, 36,6,365-374.

Meyer A The Philosophy of Occupational Therapy. (Reprinted from the Archives of Occupational Therapy, Vol 1, pp1-10) in *AJOT* 1922, 1,10,639-642, 17.

Reilly M. Occupational therapy can be one of the great ideas of 20th century medicine. *AJOT*, 1962, 16,1-9.

Reilly M. An Explanation of Play. In Reilly M.(Ed.) *Play As Exploratory Learning: Studies of Curiosity Behavior*. (Pp.117-155) Beverly Hills, CA: Sage Publications.

Rogers J. Order and Disorder in Medicine and Occupational Therapy. *AJOT*, 1982, 36,1,29-35.

White R.H. Motivation Reconsidered: The Concept of Competence. *Psychological Review*, 1959, 66, 126-134.

White R.H. Competence and the Psychosexual stages of development. Nebraska Symposium on Motivation. Lincoln: Univ. of Nebraska, 1960.

Chapter
9

An Acquisitional Approach

The acquisitional frame of reference is "the structure for linking learning theories, the reality aspects of purposeful activities and the process of acquiring specific skills needed for successful participation in the environment" (Toglia & Abreu 1983). Mosey (1981) notes that in the acquisitional frame of reference, the learning of skills necessary for participation in the community need not be done according to any developmental order or sequence. Historically, this framework has its basis in classical and operant conditioning, which use external reinforcement as the motivation for learning. However, Mosey's role acquisition approach assumes a self-direction, an urge toward competence or mastery of skills not unlike that described by RH White (1967). Theories included in this chapter are the biomechanical and rehabilitative approaches, role acquisition and cognitive rehabilitation. Some of these approaches are directed toward groups with specific disabilities, and are not appropriate for a broad spectrum of patient populations.

Basic Assumptions

A common element of all the theories cited is the focus on interaction with the external environment in the present. Current, observable behavior in the context of specific roles and activities is the major concern. The whole is considered to be the sum of its parts; therefore, behavior can be broken down into its component sub-skills for the purpose of easier learning.

Biomechanical Approach

This approach is primarily appropriate for patients who lack range of motion, strength and endurance to perform daily life tasks (Trombly 1989). The theory draws upon the kinetic principles of human movement, and its goal is to restore function. These are some of the same principles of strength and effort that are presently associated with work hardening.

The maximum motion of every joint in every possible direction is called its range of motion (ROM). Average ROMs for each joint in each direction have been calculated, so that deviation from the norm, or limitation of ROM, can be determined. There are many causes of limitation in range of motion; some are head injury, stroke, burns, fractures, arthritis and peripheral nerve injury. Range of motion is measured with a goniometer, which, when applied to the joint, determines the angle or number of degrees the joint can move. For example, the typical ROM of the elbow joint is 0-150 degrees. The ROM can be measured actively, "Lift your arm high over your head" (AROM) or passively "Let me flex and extend your shoulder" (PROM). Specific guidelines for measuring range of motion for each joint may be found in Trombly (1989).

In occupational therapy, activities are devised to encourage the patient to increase and/or maintain range of motion. Particularly in groups of patients who are at risk, such as those with arthritis, multiple sclerosis, or post head trauma or stroke, exercise "classes" to maintain/extend range of motion are common. Crafts and games can be adapted by positioning them in a way that forces the patient to reach, bend, push, pull or grasp in order to accomplish the goal. Care should be taken to plan the right amount of movement, since overestimating it can easily cause injury.

Strength

Muscle weakness is another common problem treated in occupational therapy with physical disabilities. When illness or injury results in specific muscle weakness, or when weakness can potentially cause deformity, activities can be devised to increase muscle strength. Strength can be increased in several ways. Stress is applied to a muscle or muscle group by increase in load or weight. Lifting objects of gradually increased weight will strengthen the muscles. Duration of muscle contraction also influences strength. Holding a position or lifting and holding a heavy object for longer and longer intervals can increase strength. The rate and the frequency of contraction also affect strength; faster or more frequent exercise increases strength, even when lighter weight is used. Any combination of these parameters when applied to exercise have been found to increase strength. The challenge for the OT is to find activities that can be graded in load, duration, rate and frequency, so that strength can be increased gradually and without injury. Craft activities, such as sanding wood or weaving on a loom, have traditionally been adapted to accomplish these goals. When treating in groups, work activities such as gardening and landscaping, cleaning and moving furniture or stocking shelves might accomplish the goals of increasing strength.

Endurance

Endurance refers to the length of time muscles can continue to work without becoming fatigued. A person can sustain isometric contraction equivalent to 50% of maximum voluntary contraction (MVC) up to one minute. In normal subjects, contraction time and percentage of MVC are inversely related (Trombly 1989). For example, if Sally carries a 50 lb. bag of dog food from her car up three flights of stairs to her apartment, she will need to sustain a 50% MVC for two minutes. Chances are it will be necessary for Sally to stop and rest after one minute before continuing. However, if she carries a 25 lb. bag of dog food, she can sustain a 25% MVC for the two minutes it takes her to walk all the way to her apartment without resting.

In occupational therapy, endurance may be increased by using moderately fatiguing activities for progressively longer periods of time. The OT can offer activities that sustain interest over the needed increases in duration. In the area of group treatment, many active games and sports can be adapted to the goal of increasing strength and endurance. Tug of war, for example, can be timed so that the length of effort progressively increases with each round. Relay races, perhaps carrying progressively heavier items, can be graded also.

Rehabilitative Approach

The rehabilitative approach is "a compensatory approach for patients who need to live with a disability on a temporary or permanent basis"(Trombly 1989, 3). Using this approach, the physical disability patient uses his or her remaining abilities to perform needed tasks. Occupational therapy helps to compensate for loss in order to accomplish activities of daily living.

An important aspect of the rehabilitation approach is developing patient competence in performance of occupational roles. The patient should identify the roles he or she will continue; for example, worker, spouse, club member, and friend. The roles played, in turn, help define the tasks the individual must learn or re-learn. The goals are specific, and occupational therapy treatment centers around accomplishing those specific goals or tasks which the patient has identified as his or her preferences.

The OT organizes the environment, then motivates and reinforces the patient toward successful completion of the task. Adaptations, compensations and adaptive equipment may be incorporated. Competence in doing the task is achieved through repetition and practice.

Mosey and Role Acquisition

Mosey addresses this frame of reference to those individuals whose disability has stabilized and who continue to have difficulty in performance of tasks of their major social roles (Robertson 1988). She identifies the basic skills common to all social roles as **task skills** and **interpersonal skills**. These basic skills are necessary building blocks for the performance of self-care (activities of daily living), family interaction, recreation and work. Temporal adaptation, or skill in the perception and use of time, serves to organize and balance the tasks of occupational roles on a daily basis.

The learning of tasks and social roles involves both a sociological and a psychological perspective. In socialization, the values and traditions of one's cultural background influence the learning of social roles. These roles are learned through interaction with others in a setting that demands the performance of specific social behaviors. For example, in school, the child learns to be a student by watching his peers (role models), and by following the teacher's instruction (read this story to the class). Tasks are learned through a combination of inherent capacities, attention and motivation, active participation and reinforcement or feedback.

Mosey defines the skills necessary for the major categories of function. The task skills are listed as follows:
1. willingness to engage in tasks;
2. adequate posture for tasks;
3. physical strength and endurance;

4. gross and fine motor coordination;
5. interest in task;
6. rate of performance;
7. ability to follow oral, demonstrated, pictorial and written directions;
8. use of tools and materials;
9. acceptable level of neatness;
10. attention to detail;
11. ability to solve problems;
12. ability to organize task in logical manner;
13. ability to tolerate frustration;
14. ability be self-directed.

The interpersonal skills are listed as the ability to:
1. initiate, respond to and sustain verbal interactions;
2. express ideas and feelings;
3. be aware of needs and feelings of others;
4. participate in cooperative and competitive situations;
5. compromise and negotiate;
6. assert self;
7. take on appropriate group roles.

Skills are separately defined for family interaction, activities of daily living, leisure and work. **Temporal adaptation**, the ability to perceive and manage time, is defined as orientation, organization, planning, goal setting, and establishing a schedule.

Mosey suggests that treatment in task skill development begin on an individual basis. Group treatment can be effective in learning the more advanced task skills, and in working on interpersonal skills. She suggests topical or thematic groups be designed to address specific skills. A cooking group, for example, might follow the theme of preparing meals, serving them, and socializing while eating them. The group gives members practice in doing a variety of tasks, and taking on a variety of social roles. Many of the identified skills could be incorporated into a cooking group. In this frame of reference, however, Mosey warns that groups must be carefully structured around the specific skills to be learned.

The role acquisition frame of reference can be conceptualized by the hierarchy pictured in Figure 9-1.

Denton and Functional Performance

Another theory that seems to fit in this category is Denton's "functional performance" (1987). This theory seems to summarize many of the same components mentioned earlier. Functional performance calls for the identification of problems in the performance of work, play or self-maintenance. Underlying problematic performance may be more basic problems in five component systems: sensory integration, motor, psychologic, cognitive and social functioning. Dysfunction, in Denton's view, is lack of skill, and treatment focuses on the learning of needed skills with the goal of improving function.

Cognitive Rehabilitation

This category involves the human's ability to process information. Its roots are in the neuroanatomy and neurophysiology of the brain. Some of the domains of concern include attention, perception, and problem-solving. Aleksandr Luria provides a useful organization

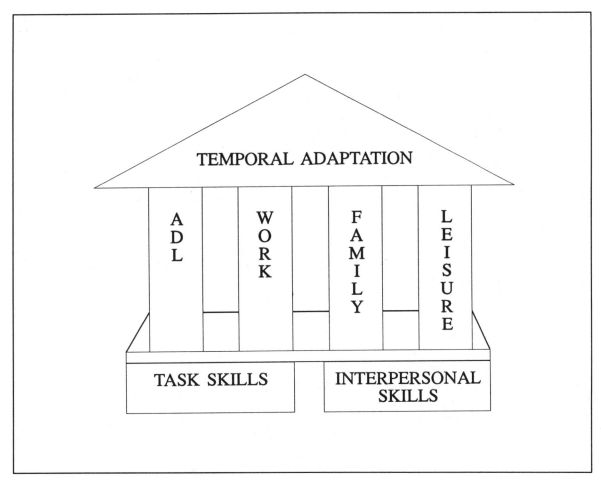

Figure 9-1. Mosey's Role Acquisition Hierarchy.

of brain function, which helps us understand how different areas and types of injury affect performance (Luria 1966). However, whether the injury produces perceptual, motor, language or perceptual deficits, the approach to treatment of these deficits is clearly acquisitional. Cognitive remediation involves a progression of exercises that provide practice in the use of specific skills. The major contributors to occupational therapy in this area will be reviewed. They are Joan Toglia and Beatrix Abreu and Claudia Allen.

Toglia and Abreu

"Learning theory is the foundation for perceptual-cognitive training" according to Toglia and Abreu (1983). This training involves systematic procedures provided to assist patients in the perception of stimuli and the effective solving of problems. The techniques presented by Toglia and Abreu use activities that are cortical in nature, techniques of cuing, generalization of learning and representational (perceptual) as well as symbolic (words and numbers) learning.

Toglia and Abreu refer to Luria's brain region classifications in their organization of perceptual and cognitive deficits. The *first* brain area described includes the brain stem and the old cortex, containing the midbrain, thalamus, hypothalamus, uncas, reticular formation and cerebellum. These are the innermost portions of the brain, and are responsible for attention, wakefulness, arousal and response to stimuli.

The *second* brain area Luria defines includes the backmost areas and is responsible for analysis, coding and storage of information. It receives raw data from sensory systems and assigns meaning to it. Luria's *third* functional area includes the frontal portions of the brain, and is responsible for intentions and programs and problem solving.

A distinction is also made between the right and left hemispheres of the brain in terms of function. The **right hemisphere** is responsible for diffuse representation, gestalts and organized wholes. It deals in concepts rather than specifics, and processes visual-spatial data and non verbal sounds. Body scheme and tactile, somato-sensory integration are primarily attributed to the right side of the brain. The **left hemisphere** is analytic and sequential, concerned with language, specific details and mathematical operations. While there are discrete characteristics for the two sides of the brain, functionally they work together to perform daily life tasks.

Luria tells us that the many parts of the brain work together to perform complex functions, therefore specific areas of the brain cannot clearly be connected with specific functions. Our knowledge of the temporal, occipital, parietal and frontal lobes of the brain as well as the right and left hemispheres does not yet explain exactly how these parts interrelate. Often, it is through clinical work with brain damaged patients that we learn what types of functions are lost when certain parts of the brain are damaged.

Accidents and illness which cause damage to discrete areas of the brain are the most likely candidates for cognitive and perceptual retraining. Luria's organization of brain function is helpful as a guide in assessing the areas of dysfunction and planning strategies for retraining. Some of the theories about how cognitive rehabilitation works are outlined by Bracy (1986) as follows:

1. Lower brain areas take control and compensate for lost skills at higher levels.
2. Different brain areas take over for or replace lost skills (opposite hemisphere, for example).
3. Normal function returns as shock effect of injury subsides.
4. Function is recovered through retraining.

According to Luria (1973), rehabilitation involves the reorganization of functional systems so that new methods of performing old behaviors are acquired. The retraining involves repetitive exercises which place demands on the individual to perform skills of graded difficulty. Compensation is applied when no further skill development in a given area appears possible.

The six basic areas of perception/cognition identified by Toglia and Abreu (1983) are orientation, attention, visual processing, motor planning, cognition and occupational behavior. All of these areas form the basis for the selection of group activities. There are numerous workbooks and collections of exercises that exist in the literature that are most helpful in planning groups. As described later, the type of group treatment best suited to this frame of reference is the parallel group, in which members do individual tasks in a side-by-side manner.

Allen

Another author who has contributed to the theory of cognitive rehabilitation is Claudia Allen. Allen's approach involves the role of cognition in the ability to perform tasks. Allen's criteria for the six cognitive levels as applied to a chronic psychiatric population appears in Chapter 5. However, her contributions to the theory of cognitive cuing, activity analysis and task equivalence are useful guidelines for the development of groups in cognitive rehabilitation of physically disabled patients as well. Allen (1987) states that the thoughts that guide purposeful actions are formed by associating a sensory cue with a motor action. The cuing that will be effective changes with each cognitive level (refer to Chapter 5, Table 5-1). Here is a summary:

Level 1 – subliminal cues, patient attends to internal stimuli primarily (hunger, pain), difficult to get patient's attention at all;

Level 2 – uses movement or proprioceptive cues, the body's comfort is the basis of response;

Level 3 – uses tactile cues, touching the patient will capture his attention, patient can repeat an action but does not generalize;

Level 4 – uses visual cues, patient can learn by watching a demonstration, or looking at a finished product;

Level 5 – uses trial and error to learn, patient can be told or shown what to do, and can generalize learning to new situations;

Level 6 – involves planning, reflection and anticipation and cues in the form of abstract ideas or symbols (reading) can be utilized.

Cues at these six levels are valuable to the occupational therapist in understanding how a patient can learn new skills. Practice and therapeutic cuing at the appropriate level can maximize the effectiveness of the patient in performing tasks. Allen also emphasizes the importance of the environment in planning activity groups for patients at different cognitive levels. Availability of materials and assistance are defined at each level (see Chapter 5).

A related scale that is useful in assessing levels of cognitive functioning is the head trauma levels developed at Rancho Los Amigos Hospital (Trombly 1989). These describe the levels of reaction to stimuli or response to the environment.

Level I – no response, unresponsive to stimuli;

Level II – generalized response, non-specific, inconsistent and non-purposeful reaction to stimuli;

Level III – localized response, response directly related to type of stimuli, yet still inconsistent and delayed;

Level IV – confused, agitated, response heightened, severely confused and could be bizarre;

Level V – confused, inappropriate, some response to simple commands but confusion with the more complex commands, high level of distractibility;

Level VI – confused, appropriate, response more goal directed, but cues necessary;

Level VII – automatic, appropriate, response robot-like, judgment and problem-solving lacking;

Level VIII – purposeful, appropriate, response adequate, subtle deficits persist.

These levels are somewhat parallel to Allen's levels, but begin at a lower level, so the numbers do not correspond. Both of these scales give occupational therapists guidelines for forming groups of patients at similar levels and planning appropriate activities and learning strategies.

Function and Dysfunction

Function in the acquisitional frame of reference refers simply to the successful performance of the skills necessary to work, play/leisure, self-care and social roles.

Dysfunction is the lack of skills to perform these roles. The emphasis is placed on concrete, observable behavior. Mosey outlines seven continuums of function and dysfunction: task skills, interpersonal skills, family interaction, activities of daily living, school or work, play/leisure/recreation and temporal adaptation. Skills or the lack of skills in each of these areas determines function and dysfunction (Mosey 1988). Toglia and Abreu look at brain functioning as the behavior to be measured, and measure this by the outward manifestations of orientation, attention, visual processing, motor planning, cognition (memory, organization and problem-solving) and occupational behavior (Toglia and Abreu 1987). Allen's conception is similar to this; her view of competence is measured by attention, conscious awareness and motor actions in the performance of tasks (Allen 1985, 1992).

Change and Motivation

Following the guidelines of learning theory and behavior modification, the basic strategy for change is reinforcement. Change occurs when the correct behavior is observed by the therapist and reinforced in some way. The type of reinforcement that can be effective will vary from patient to patient. Some patients do not seem to have the internal motivation to learn new skills. For these patients, external reward is most appropriate. This can be anything the patient is willing to work for, such as praise, extra attention, candy, cigarettes or privileges. Some patients respond to social reinforcement, such as the praise and acceptance of their peers, family or friends. At a higher level, patients will strive to learn skills or improve functioning in order to gain the approval of society, or meet the expectations of their cultural group.

In Mosey's "role acquisition" frame, intrinsic motivation is assumed. Change will occur through successful experiences in the mastery of skills. In occupational therapy, simple skills are mastered before more difficult ones are attempted. Thus the patients can develop a feeling of competence as each new skill is mastered. The feeling of competence gained from successful occupational performance, in itself, provides reinforcement. This is known as self-reinforcement, the highest form of motivation patients can achieve.

Group Treatment

Role of the Occupational Therapist

In many ways, the manner of leadership in the acquisitional frame is similar to the psychoeducational model. The therapist is essentially a directive leader, the resident expert in the group. The relationship is similar to the teacher-student relationship, with specific lessons and strategies for teaching them designed by the therapist and presented to the group. The group itself is designed as a parallel group, with patients learning new skills side-by-side. Interaction is not generally expected or necessary. Certain types of interaction, however, should be encouraged. Patients learning to cope with disability are often able to provide needed support and feedback to one another. This feedback can serve as part of the learning as well as reinforcing correct responses. The occupational therapist should carefully monitor the interaction in these groups, however, to make sure the feedback given is of a helpful and therapeutic nature.

Designing groups in this frame is especially important. Careful assessment of patients prior to assigning them to groups will ensure that the members are compatible and can reinforce each other while learning. Groups in this frame are primarily homogeneous. They are grouped because of a common need to learn a particular skill. They should be at approximately the same level cognitively, so that they will be able to learn at the same pace, and through similar modes of presentation. Groups working on perception and memory skills, for example, might be given several memory games during a therapy session. All the members should be able to understand the verbal directions if the activity is to be successful in accomplishing its goal.

Heterogeneous groups are also workable in this frame of reference, but they are more difficult to plan for and manage. For example, patients with different physical problems, may be able to work together to accomplish tasks that none could do alone. A baking group might consist of orthopedic, hemiplegic and arthritic patients, all of whom might be assigned different parts of the task. The orthopedic patient might only be able to read the recipe, the arthritic patients could gather ingredients, while the hemiplegic patient does the mixing. All of these patients' goals might be different, but they could all benefit from the experience of working together.

Goals

The goal in the acquisitional frame of reference, is to demonstrate improvement in functional performance. In working directly with physical or cognitive/perceptual dysfunction, the therapist may set the goal, based on her best assessment of the patient's potential. Norms are helpful in setting goals in the biomechanical areas, i.e.,"resume normal strength in an injured leg"..."work up to two hours before rest." In a patient with temporary cognitive impairment, Allen's level 6 or Rancho's level VIII, may be an appropriate goal.

However, when dealing with the rehabilitation of occupational roles, the patient's own values and preferences often determine the goal. Long term goals may be set based on the patient's expected environment (Mosey 1988). In this case, goals are set collaboratively with the patient and activities are chosen based on his or her interests and preferences.

In planning group treatment, patients with similar needs or deficits are usually grouped together, and goals are set to address their common deficiencies. For example, in a problem-solving group, the goals might be to master each step in the problem-solving process. Patients will be able to:

1. clearly state the desired outcome of the problem;
2. gather relevant information;
3. analyze and interpret the data;
4. devise a plan to solve the problem (describe the actions that need to be taken, and sequence the steps);
5. implement the plan;
6. evaluate the outcome.

The goals in the acquisitional frame of reference are always very specific, observable and measurable. This is because the treatment approach is very goal-directed. The activities used are designed to accomplish specific goals. This principle is very important to keep in mind when planning groups using the acquisitional frame of reference.

Examples of Activities

The following are some examples of activities that are designed to accomplish specific acquisitional goals.

Exercise Groups

Exercise to music or dance activities have good potential as therapeutic tools. Circle or group dancing is usually best suited to our purpose in occupational therapy. In physical disability areas where goals involve maintaining and increasing strength and range of motion, group activities that accomplish these goals are more enjoyable and motivating than individual exercise programs. A good example of this type of group is the "Range of Motion Dance," an exercise program for patients with rheumatoid arthritis developed by Diane Harlowe and Patricia Yu at St. Mary's Hospital Medical Center in Madison, Wisconsin (Van Deusen & Harlowe, 1987). This is a guided fantasy done with groups of arthritis patients seated in chairs. The exercises, while following the story, go systematically through the range of motion for nearly every joint in the body. Once the sequence of motions is learned, it can be repeated by the patients at home by listening to the story on an audiotape. Greenfield and Godinez have introduced a similar group for stroke patients, called "self-range-of-motion (SROM) exercises" (1989). They have defined eight skill levels for these exercises, ranging from complete dependence on the therapist leader to independence in performing the exercises.

In doing such groups, it is important to use the potential of the group to provide mutual support, encouragement and feedback. Don't let the activity speak for itself; combine it with verbal reinforcement, progress checks and education about how and why it's helping. It is generally the social and emotional aspects of a group that keep members coming back.

Map Reading

A group of cognitively impaired patients has the goal of improving skills in visual perception and verbal communication. They are given a map of their community, and a worksheet with a list of ten locations. Their tasks are to:

1. Write directions from Merritt Parkway to the Trumbull Shopping Mall on Main Street.
2. Write directions from the corner of Madison and Stonehouse Roads to Trumbull High School on Stroebel and Daniels Farms Roads.
3. Describe two alternate routes to get from the golf course on Tashua Road to Main Street at the Bridgeport line.
4. Direct someone from Teller and Whitney to the dog pound on Church Street.
5. Plan a route to pick up three friends, on Indian Ledge Road, Brittany Road, and Autumn Ridge Road and take them to the Town Hall meeting room on Quality Street.

Other locations can be added, and directions given verbally or in writing. Each patient in the group should have at least one location to find on his own, and then communicate the directions to the rest of the group. The therapist should encourage members to give each other feedback about the accuracy of the directions and clarity of communication.

Design Duplication

This activity appears in *The Cognitive Rehabilitation Workbook* by Dougherty and Radomski (1987). The goals are to give and follow verbal directions. The objectives are to develop vocabulary to give concise directions, increase accuracy in conveying detailed information, and develop a tolerance for the pitfalls in making oneself understood. Followers of directions are expected to increase their accuracy, develop skills in clarification and confirmation and increase speed of processing verbal directions.

A group of six is divided into pairs. One from each pair acts as the direction giver and holds a line drawing of several lines and shapes. The other half of each pair sits with his back to his partner and holds a clipboard with blank paper and a pencil with an eraser. Both partners are provided with rulers. Partner 1 must verbally describe the line drawing so that partner 2 can draw an exact duplicate of the drawing being described. Attention must be paid to shapes, spacing and dimensions. The pair has 20 minutes to accomplish the task. Then a new drawing is given to each pair and roles are reversed.

It is very important that a feedback session follow each trial. The pairs should discuss the results and analyze any errors in communication in order to correct these on the next trial. This activity can be fun as well as useful, and the therapist should try to create a relaxed atmosphere for the group.

Group Leadership

Introduction

The groups in this framework vary from very low to very high cognitive functioning. Therefore the explanation of purpose in acquisitional groups needs to be adapted to fit the patients' level of cognitive understanding. In groups with physical disabilities and normal cognitive functioning it is especially important to explain the purpose thoroughly. The purpose of different techniques in treatment and the reason for application of certain activities becomes part of the patient's overall education about his disability and allows his participation in developing coping strategies. Discussing therapist expectations for progress or the rate of progress will prevent patients from having unrealistically high expectations and then feeling they have failed when they cannot achieve them. For example, a group may be given a memory exercise of remembering objects, and repeating them back five minutes later. Patients with memory impairment should understand that they are not failures if they can't remember all items. Explaining the time frame: "You will be asked to remember these objects after 5 minutes, 10 minutes, 20 minutes and 40 minutes." will give patients an opportunity to apply compensatory strategies, and to establish self-expectations.

A warm-up is not always necessary in acquisitional groups. When appropriate, a warm-up is used to size up the group. By giving the group a shorter, simpler version of the main event, the therapist can preview patient performance and adapt the activity accordingly. For example, in the design duplication activity described earlier, a single straight line design across the paper might be given as a warm-up. This simple activity allows patients to practice the format of sitting back to back, verbally describing the line drawing, using the ruler, and attempting to replicate the line with verbal instruction. Success with this simple activity also prepares patients psychologically for attempting more difficult designs.

Activity

The length of time spent in doing the activity is longer than in most other frames of reference. At least two thirds of the session is spent on the activity itself. The occupational therapist chooses an activity for its potential to facilitate the acquisition of skills. Each activity should be thoroughly prepared with precise verbal instructions, demonstrations and examples as appropriate. Worksheets, pencils, calculators, rulers or whatever materials are needed should be available for each patient, and sharing of these should be minimized.

Activity selection can be very challenging for the therapist, because it requires a nearly exact match between the patient's ability and the task demand. Patients can be very easily discouraged when presented with tasks that are beyond their capabilities. Guidelines such as Allen's cognitive levels or Rancho's head trauma levels are useful for planning activities that are within a patient's ability. A description of Allen's level 4, for example, tells us that it will be necessary to demonstrate the steps of a task, and that a sample of the completed project provides the necessary visual cues. A unique feature of groups in this frame of reference is the necessity of assisting patients in completing the activity. Toglia and Abreu (1987) offer some helpful treatment principles for cuing:

1. Direct to where task or activity begins, using visual, auditory and kinesthetic cues.
2. Direct client where to look, increase client's visual scanning ability.
3. Direct client in adjusting his speed of response to match and succeed...bring awareness if he is going too fast or too slow.
4. Direct client in adjusting focus to stimulus event frequency.
5. Restructure and reorganize non-human environment
6. Assist client in identifying his perceptual strategies
7. Select activities or tasks that have individual motivational forces.
8. Provide feedback
   a. correction, explanation of behavior
   b. reinforcement.

The process of cuing continues from therapist to each group member throughout the activity. This requires the OT to take an active role in providing not only the activity instructions and materials, but also encouragement, support and feedback. This kind of leadership can be exhausting for the therapist. Therefore, when patients are likely to need constant cuing and direction, groups should be kept small.

The environment is another important aspect of the activity. The setting should be arranged to enhance the learning potential of the group members. Factors that may cause distraction, such as extremes of heat or cold, too little or too much light, extraneous noise and clutter, should be eliminated. Arranging of chairs, tables and materials should be done before the group begins. Sometimes patients who arrive early can help with this process, but not to the extent that their involvement detracts from their participation in the activity.

The therapist puts great thought into arranging an optimum learning environment. Sometimes objects are deliberately set out to provide stimulation and challenge. For example, the use of pocket calculators in a cognitive exercise involving math calculations can provide the needed motivation for patients to perform an otherwise boring or unliked task. The use of music in exercise groups performs a similar function.

The directions for an activity, like the purpose in the introduction, should be tailored to the group's cognitive ability to understand them. All of the sensory systems can be utilized in communicating the directions: verbal instruction, visual illustration or demonstration, or touching and moving the patient through a specified motor sequence. Perceptual training may involve other types of stimuli, such as taste or smell as well.

Sharing and Processing

Patients often do activities individually within an acquisitional group. How much is shared, depends on the learning potential of the sharing. In a problem-solving group, members may benefit from sharing their creative solutions. A group learning to use adaptive equipment may find little benefit in sharing. A discussion of feelings about an activity may be helpful in giving one another emotional support. The therapist needs to decide how much mutual support is desirable to the group before planning discussion questions that encourage it. The emphasis in the acquisitional frame of reference is on the learning of skills, and discussion of other issues must be evaluated as they relate to this learning.

A certain amount of process discussion, that focuses on how members relate to one another, can enhance patient motivation to learn more. Interaction has potential to put members at ease, and to emotionally prepare them for learning. Often in groups with physical disabilities, occupational therapists seem to ignore the normal group developmental process that all groups experience. Relationships between members don't always end up being positive; often patients in a group can distract or even annoy one another. This calls for therapist intervention to prevent the negative interactions from detracting from group learning. A process illumination, in which the therapist shares his/her awareness of group theory, may be appropriate in helping the group resolve interpersonal conflicts. Allowing the members to express feelings about one another, and having them acknowledged by the therapist, may clear the air considerably, even though there is no immediate resolution. It is not an expectation, in acquisitional groups, that members like each other. It is only necessary that they can work together to accomplish the therapeutic goal.

Generalizing and Application

The generalizations derived from the group should never stray too far from the goals. This part of the group discussion is usually led by the therapist. How the responses of the members were alike or different, may not even be relevant. The desired outcome of learning skills in the clinic, is that they be generalized to the patient's expected environment after discharge. A discussion of *how* they might be generalized to specific situations in their home environment leads nicely into application. Many of the books and articles on techniques appropriate to the acquisitional frame of reference, refer to the lack of efficacy research. Whether or not the practice exercises done in the occupational therapy clinic are likely to result in greater independence in occupational functioning, is always under question. However, an open group discussion about how the skills learned in therapeutic groups can apply to each patient, may make this more likely to occur. If the patients are consciously aware of the usefulness of certain skills, they may communicate this to family members and caretakers, and they may initiate the process of self-reinforcement.

Summary

A verbal summary by the therapist is a tradition to be continued throughout the frames of reference. In this one, its major purpose is to reinforce learning. Emphasizing the important points of the session, and giving positive feedback to members are the important elements. The few minutes it takes to summarize, may make the difference between forgetting and remembering what was learned.

Bibliography

Allen C. *Occupational Therapy for Psychiatric Diseases: Measurement and Management of Cognitive Disabilities.* Boston/Toronto: Little Brown, 1985.

Allen C. and Earhart K. *OT Treatment Goals for the Physically and Cognitively Disabled.* Rockville, MD: AOTA, 1992.

Bracy O. Cognitive rehabilitation: A process approach. *J Cognitive Rehabilitation*, Mar/Apr, 10-17, 1986.

David S. Allen cognitive level and sensorimotor treatment in acute care. *Sensory Integration SIS Newsletter*, 11, 1, 1-3 (AOTA) 1988.

Dougherty P. and Radomski MV. *The Cognitive Rehabilitation Workbook.* Rockville, MD: Aspen, 1987.

Luria A. *The Working Brain.* NY: Basic Books, 1973.

Luria A. *Higher Cortical Functions in Man. NY: Basic Books, 1966.*

Mosey AC. 1988. Role acquisition: An acquisitional frame of reference, in Robertson S. *Mental Health Focus*, Rockville, Md., AOTA, 1988.

Toglia J. and Abreu B. *Cognitive Rehabilitation.* NY, authors, 1987. (J.Toglia, New York Hospital, 525 E 68th St. Room 1826, New York, NY 10021).

Trombly C. *Occupational Therapy for Physical Dysfunction.* 3rd ed. Baltimore, Williams & Wilkins, 1989.

Van Deusen J. and Harlowe D. The efficacy of the ROM dance program for adults with rheumatoid arthritis. *AJOT*, 41,2,90-95, 1987.

White RH. Competence and the growth of personality. (in Science and Psychoanalysis, Vol. XI, The Ego, NY: Grune and Stratton, 1967).

SECTION THREE

Planning an Occupational Therapy Group

Introduction

The final step in the learning process of occupational therapy group treatment is applying our knowledge to patient populations. Chapters 10 and 11 take the form of guided learning experiences. Chapter 10, *Writing a Group Treatment Protocol*, gives guidelines for thinking about the needs of a patient population within a frame of reference, and generating a written group plan.

One of the keys to successful application of theory lies in the understanding of patient dysfunction. It has been pointed out that the parts of function and dysfunction that are addressed changes in each frame of reference. In addition, it is important to remember that function and dysfunction are very different from diagnosis. Diagnosis is a medical term which identifies illness and guides medical treatment. Occupational therapy's emphasis on a patient's adaptive function looks beyond diagnosis to the consequence of illness and disease with regard to everyday activities.

In Chapter 10, the group planning process begins with an analysis of the patient population to be treated. This is a reality-oriented approach which looks at some of the typical treatment settings where OTs work. As the occupational therapist assesses the patient population for which group activities will be designed, he/she must look carefully at the consequences of illness in terms of impairments, disabilities and handicaps. The World Health Organization's (WHO) 1980 publication, *International Classification of Impairments, Disabilities and Handicaps* is a helpful guide to our understanding of patient dysfunction. WHO defines impairment in the context of health as a loss or abnormality of psychological, physiological or anatomical structure or function. Disability, in the context of health experience, is any restriction or lack of ability to perform an activity in the manner or within the range considered normal for a human being. A handicap is a disadvantage for a given individual, resulting from an impairment or a disability, that limits or prevents fulfillment of a role that is normal (depending on age, sex and cultural factors) for that individual. A disability is considered within the context of the person, while a handicap relates to society or compliance with social norms. This distinction helps the occupational therapist to address the consequences of illness that can be best affected through group activities.

Chapter 11, *A Group Laboratory Experience*, offers a group membership experience as a context for learning about group dynamics. This chapter follows the guidelines of Chapter 10 and provides an example of the analysis of the needs of a student population. *Developing Your Professional Self* is an example of a group protocol which can be beneficial for students' professional development as they approach the clinical training phase of their education. In the five years we have been doing these groups for second semester juniors, the feedback from students has been excellent. In addition to learning and applying the principles of group dynamics, students have found the feedback for themselves invaluable for their own professional growth.

These two experiences should facilitate the application of theory in practice. The process of this text has gone from concrete (the format), to abstract (the frames) and then back to concrete (the plan). This is not unlike the clinical reasoning process itself, which swings back and forth between the empirical and the hypothetical as the therapy process progresses. A good group plan involves the empirical collection of data about patients' impairments, disabilities and handicaps, the formation of a hypothesis about what kind of group activity might be helpful and method for evaluation of treatment outcome after implementation (empirical again). The laboratory experience for students demonstrates this process.

Finally, as part of the practical application of theory to the group planning process, the student is encouraged to think about how the original seven step format changes with each frame of reference. As a learning guide, a chart comparing group leadership in the seven frames of reference is presented in Appendix E.

Bibliography

World Health Organization International Classification of Impairments, Disabilities and Handicaps, 1980. Distributed by Q Corp., 49 Sheridan Ave., Albany, NY.

Chapter
10

Writing A Group
Treatment Protocol

The group protocol is an extensive and detailed outline of a group to be planned by the occupational therapist for a specific patient population. This exercise is intended to prepare therapists to plan effective programs to meet the needs of patients in a wide variety of diagnostic categories, and using a variety of frames of reference. Several steps have been outlined to clarify our clinical thinking about groups. They are: identifying a patient population, selecting a frame of reference, selecting what aspect of treatment to address, writing a group treatment outline and planning individual sessions.

Identifying Your Patient Population

For the purposes of learning, the student should choose one of the following treatment settings where occupational therapists typically treat patients. This will be the patient population around which you will plan your group. Use the Patient Population Worksheet to help you.
- Long-term adolescent mental health institute
- Twenty-eight day inpatient adult substance abuse program
- Stroke recovery unit
- Chronic mental illness ward
- Unit for traumatic brain injured adults
- Group home for adults with developmental disabilities
- Outpatient program for adults with physical disability

- Geriatrics, nursing home care
- Acute adult psychiatric ward (average stay 2-4 weeks)
- Hand injury clinic

Settings should be chosen on the basis of interest, prior experience or curiosity. The planning will incorporate a process of familiarization with the chosen population. Since most students do not have much experience, it is advisable to contact a local treatment center and arrange a visit. Fieldwork I experience or prior volunteer experience is also helpful. It is impossible to plan an effective group treatment experience without some knowledge of the population for which it is intended.

Another way to become more familiar with the population you choose is to do some reference reading. Many excellent books are available describing specific diagnostic categories, such as Alzheimer's disease, multiple sclerosis, drug abuse, eating disorders and mental retardation. Reading case studies of people with these disorders is particularly helpful.

Probably the most motivating way to choose a diagnostic category is personal experience. Many students have friends or relatives who may have a disorder that fits one of the listed categories. Writing a group protocol for a specific individual and others with the same disorder gives the student the advantage of greater personal understanding. It may be easier to imagine the impact of certain group activities, and the barriers that may need to be addressed.

Patient Population Worksheet

1. Population choice
Choose a treatment setting from those listed on the previous pages. If you like more than one, list "pros" and "cons" of each to help you decide.

First choice _____

    pros: 1   cons: 1

             2   2

             3   3

Second choice _____

    pros: 1   cons: 1

             2   2

             3   3

2. Population definition

    a. Identify two centers nearby that treat this population.

        Center _____ telephone # _____

        Address _____

        Contact person/therapist _____

        Center _____ telephone # _____

        Address _____

        Contact person/therapist _____

    b. Describe patient characteristics typical of the center.

        Age range _____ male/female/both _____

        Diagnostic categories _____

        _____

        _____

        Patients' education level _____

        Patients' living arrangement when not hospitalized _____

        _____

        _____

        Occupation/work status _____

        _____

        Socioeconomic status _____

Patient Population Worksheet (continued)

c. Predict rehabilitation potential

Approximate level of functioning (high, medium, low) _____

Describe _____

Physical limitations _____

_____

Verbal ability/interaction potential _____

_____

Probable discharge plan _____

_____

d. Describe treatment setting

Type of treatment setting (day treatment, inpatient, clinic) _____

_____

Treatment setting's frame of reference (if known) _____

_____

How to Select a Frame of Reference

After you describe your patient population, the next decision to make is what frame of reference to use. There are several factors to consider in this decision. The preceding seven chapters can be consulted for a better understanding of the choices. While there are many frames of references in occupational therapy, for this assignment, try to stick with one of the seven included in this text. While personal beliefs usually have some influence over frame of reference selection, students should become competent in using all of them.

The major factor in the selection should be what is likely to work best for the patient. Sometimes the treatment setting has an identified frame of reference, and if so, the occupational therapist should find an occupational therapy frame of reference that is compatible with it. Some helpful factors to consider are: view of function and dysfunction, patient physical and cognitive level of function, change strategies, view of motivation, treatment time frame and treatment options.

Definition of Function and Dysfunction

Each frame of reference has its unique point of view of disability. Looking at your patient population, compare their abilities and disabilities with the explanations of function and dysfunction given in each frame of reference. Which frame best explains the function and dysfunction you see in your patients? Why?

_____

_____

_____

_____

Patient Level of Functioning

Some frames of reference have a greater usefulness for higher functioning patients, while some relate better to lower levels of functioning. Which frame offers treatment guidelines that have been effective for your patients' level of functioning? Summarize guidelines given to your patients.

_____

_____

_____

_____

Change Strategies

Another way the frames of reference differ is in their view of the change process. Some depend on the therapeutic relationship or on group interaction to facilitate change, while others rely more heavily on the components of tasks and activities, or on the environment. Think about what changes your patients need to make. Then look at the explanations given by the frames of reference on how change takes place. Which do you think might work the best for your patients? Why?

_____

_____

_____

_____

How to Select a Frame of Reference (Continued)

Motivation

How motivated are your patients? What forces do you think might motivate them to make positive changes? Each frame of reference explains motivation differently. The existential/humanistic view is freedom from anxiety and self-actualization. The ego adaptive, developmental and neurophysiological frames of reference and model of human occupation describe a drive toward mastery, but each defines something different to be mastered. The cognitive behavioral approach looks at various forms of reinforcement as the motivator. The goals of most of our occupational therapy groups are to help patients achieve a higher level of function or adaptation. However, it is not enough for the therapist to be motivated. We need to think about our patients' motivation as well. Which frame of reference best explains how our patients could be motivated? Why?

_____

_____

_____

_____

Treatment Time Frame

Some frames of reference work best for long-term treatment that encourages the development of relationships and insight, while others lend themselves to more immediate goals. For the purposes of this assignment, the treatment runs for six sessions of one hour each. But these could be spread out once a week for six weeks or condensed into two sessions a day for three days. If there is no center mentioned, what would be the most likely setting for the patient population you have chosen? Acute settings can be assumed to average ten days to two weeks. Substance abuse programs are generally three to four weeks of intensive inpatient treatment. Day treatment can go on for a year or more and chronic conditions can be treated for a lifetime. How long are your patients likely to be in treatment? Which frame of reference best fits the time frame at your identified treatment center?

_____

_____

_____

_____

Treatment Options

Each frame of reference has different guidelines for activity selection. Some have specific suggestions, while others are more flexible and able to be adapted. Look at the options suggested by the frame of reference and decide which would most interest you and your patients. Which frame of reference offers treatment options that would interest you? What are they? Which frame of reference offers treatment options that would interest your patients and/or best meet their needs? What are some options you might choose?

_____

_____

_____

_____

Selecting What Aspect of Treatment to Address

All of the occupational performance areas and occupational components which make up the domain of concern of occupational therapy have been listed and organized in one convenient document. That document is called *Uniform Terminology for Occupational Therapy,* written and revised in April 1989 by the American Occupational Therapy Association. The revised 2nd edition is reprinted in Appendix D of this text. This document was published in December 1989 in the American Occupational Therapy Journal, along with a guide for its use by Dunn and McGourty (1989). The occupational performance areas listed are activities of daily living and work activities and play or leisure activities. Activities of daily living are the following: grooming, oral hygiene, bathing, toilet hygiene, dressing, feeding and eating, medication routine, socialization, functional communication, functional mobility and sexual expression. Work activities include home management, care of others, educational and vocational activities. Play or leisure activities include both exploration and performance.

Performance components in Uniform Terminology are: sensorimotor, including sensory integration, neuromuscular and motor skills. Cognitive components include level of arousal, orientation, recognition, attention span, memory, sequencing, categorization, concept formation, intellectual operations in space, problem-solving and learning. Psychosocial skills and psychological components include psychological, social and self-management areas.

The best strategy is to go over the document in Appendix D and decide what performance areas and/or components your patients most need to work on or improve. Most patients have more than one, and activities in occupational therapy can be designed to address several of these areas or components. After looking over the document, list ten performance areas and/or components that your patient population may need to work on. In the next section, these identified aspects of treatment can help us to formulate goals for our group.

1. _____

2. _____

3. _____

4. _____

5. _____

6. _____

7. _____

8. _____

9. _____

10. _____

Group Treatment Plan Outline

Once the patient population is chosen and the frame of reference and aspects of treatment have been identified, the next step is to write a general outline. The outline should include all the factors inherent in designing a group. The general outline includes the following headings:

Group title
Author
Frame of reference
Purpose
Group membership and size
Group goals and rationale
Outcome criteria
Method
Time and place of meeting
Supplies and cost
References

This outline is intended to include not only the ingredients of an effective group treatment protocol, but also factors which will be of interest to administrators. Often occupational therapists are asked to present a group protocol to administrators prior to implementation. Administrators will need to consider factors such as group size, space, scheduling and cost. The plan you present must not only be therapeutically sound, but also cost effective.

Group Title

The name of a group is often the patient's first impression of the role occupational therapy will play in treatment. Choose it with care. Not only should a title accurately reflect the goals and content of the group, but it should also attract the patient's interest. Some examples of good titles are: "Developing Self Identity" (a group for substance abusing adolescents), "Art for Social Skills" (a group for persons with chronic mental illness) and "Re-entering Your Kitchen" (a group for postoperative cardiac patients).

Author

This includes your name and professional title: Jane Doe, OTS.

Frame of Reference

State the frame of reference you have decided to use to guide your approach to patients, organization of treatment groups and selection of activities. A single sentence on why this frame of reference is appropriate will suffice. For example: "The cognitive-behavioral approach has been widely used with substance abuse patients, and it seems to help them change their own behavior by learning new ways of thinking about their lives."

Purpose

The purpose of the group is the group's general intent. Overall goals of the group should be stated, as well as the general nature of the activities to be used. This section should be short, preferably no longer than three sentences summarizing the overall scope of the group plan. For example, the purpose of a leisure planning group might be to assist patients whose disability requires a loss of the worker role, to identify and plan for leisure activities to meet their social and emotional needs. Patients will complete written exercises, participate in group discussions and plan and carry out individual leisure activities as part of group requirements.

Group Membership and Size

The patient population for which your group is intended should be described in as much detail as possible. Not only general diagnostic factors, but factors like age, functional level, gender and role identity might be included. For purposes of referral, both inclusionary and exclusionary criteria should be described here. Inclusionary criteria describes characteristics which are appropriate for your group; exclusionary describes characteristics which are not appropriate. Some activities are appropriate for specific groups only, while others encompass a wide variety of characteristics. A target population should always be identified to give the group a focus. Broader applicability of the protocol should be described in a separate paragraph.

For the purposes of this assignment, the size of groups will be limited to three to eight members. It is generally not cost effective to treat groups of less than three and not effective treatment for more than eight. The size of a group will depend on many factors, such as the degree of impairment, the need for individual attention and the complexity of the tasks, to name a few. Group membership may be open or closed. A closed group includes all the same patients at every session for the duration of the group. An open group allows members to be added or dropped from session to session. It is generally easier to plan for closed groups, since the membership is predictable and a sense of belonging is developed. Open groups are more practical for most treatment settings and are a necessity in acute settings where patients come and go rapidly. This assignment requires you to plan a closed group. This allows the student to plan specific sessions without having to adapt to unexpected changes in membership.

Group Goals and Rationale

The goals of a group are the specific treatment aims that are intended to be met by individuals participating in the group. No less than three and no more than eight goals should be stated. Less than three usually means that goals are too vague and therefore not useful in planning specific activities. More than eight gives the group too broad a focus. Ideally, there should be at least one specific goal for each individual session planned. However, since there is usually overlap, i.e., more than one goal met with any given activity, the exact number will vary.

Goals should be stated in measurable terms. They should state what the patient will do, i.e., define, discuss, report, demonstrate. Vague terms like "learn, understand and develop" should be avoided; "attend" and "participate" are generally not enough of a description to be meaningful.

Well-written goals are the backbone of any well-designed group. They will make the rest of the group easier to plan and the outcome easier to measure. For example, the goals of a money management group might be:
1. Recognize the need for a budget.
2. List monthly income and expenses.

3. Demonstrate ability to follow a budget for one week.
4. Demonstrate specific banking skills.
5. List anticipated needs and expenses.
6. Practice comparative shopping techniques and skills to reduce impulse buying.

Once these goals are identified, the activities used to reach the goals will logically follow. Perhaps each group session can focus on a different goal, or several sessions can include more than one goal. For example, goal #4 can be addressed by giving each patient samples of a check register, check, deposit slip and withdrawal slip. Simple addition and subtraction can be practiced and included when appropriate. Use of a banking machine or telephone banking can be taught and practiced. The outcome of this activity can be measured by examining the completed forms and watching the demonstrated procedures. Specific activities and measured outcomes should follow logically from each stated goal. Rationale for goal selection should relate goals to the chosen patient population and its inherent problems. This section should explain why the goals you selected are appropriate. Limitations of the group should be mentioned—for which patients are these goals inappropriate? For example, patients who will be institutionalized may not need the skills. Precautions that may need to be taken should also be mentioned in the rationale. Adaptations that can be made to make the group useful to a wider variety of patients, perhaps in settings other than the target setting, should be mentioned here as well. For example, in the case of the money management group, the same goals can be applied to any group of patients with the goal of living independently.

Outcome Criteria

The desired results of the group should be stated in behavioral terms. By the end of the group, each patient should be able to show how he/she has progressed. The therapist needs to develop a measurable way to demonstrate the effectiveness of the group to the patient, the administrator and to those responsible for payment of services. Specific procedures should be outlined, such as a pre and post questionnaire or a pre-post rating scale for each patient. An appropriate assessment tool can be identified, if one exists, or evaluation can be specific for the group offered. If verbal feedback is used, the therapist should specify where and how this information is to be recorded. A pre-post test, assessment, questionnaire or documentation worksheet (such as the Group Member Progress Rating) must accompany your group outline as a separate sheet.

Method

An outline of the **media** to be used and the kind of **leadership** offered are key elements here. Media can be as simple as structured discussions and as complex as learning to build a small engine. Most activities are fair game. However, complex media which require special training, such as biofeedback, systematic desensitization, bioenergetics and psychodrama, should not be used. Therapeutic interventions which are the traditional roles of other disciplines, such as family therapy, unstructured verbal psychotherapy or dietary planning, should also be avoided.

The kind of leadership offered depends upon the therapist's frame of reference. If a psychoeducational format is used, the therapist may include short lecturettes on skills to be learned. (The therapist's frame of reference will determine the type of introduction and explanation given to patients during each session.) The group protocol should reflect a **consistent** frame of reference. If a humanistic or an ego adaptive approach is used, more emphasis may be placed on group interaction. Cognitive groups for lower level patients require more structured environments with carefully planned therapist assistance.

Time and Place of Meeting

Several design elements should be described in this section. For the purposes of this assignment, the time will be limited to six sessions of one hour each. The scheduling of sessions will vary according to the treatment setting. Chronic settings will accommodate weekly sessions. Acute settings may require daily meetings. The length of sessions will vary with patient attention span and type of activity chosen.

The place of meeting should be chosen with specific requirements in mind. In an actual treatment setting, a room can be identified. For the purposes of this assignment, only the characteristics of the setting should be described. The following environmental factors could be included:

- size of room
- contents - tables, chairs, cabinets, sink, etc.
- lighting, windows
- visual factors (bare walls or more home-like)
- door opened or closed
- noise factors (not next to gym or bathroom)
- accessibility of medical assistance - special telephone equipment needed, if any (kitchen for cooking activities)
- availability of assistance from therapist
- safety factors

This assignment will not limit any of these factors. A good room description will take into consideration the characteristics of the patient population chosen, as well as the activities to be included.

Supplies and Cost

The sum total of all materials and supplies and their total cost is listed here. It is recognized that copies of forms and paper and pencils or pens are generally available in most settings at no cost. Items other than these should be listed. If specific items such as videotapes or assessment materials are to be used, the name and address of the source of these should also be listed. This section will probably have to be done after specific sessions are outlined.

References

List all references that were used to create the material for the group sessions, including lecturettes, forms to be used as work sheets and other copyrighted materials. References should use the format of the American Psychological Association (1983).

Books
Author, date, title, publisher, place of publication.

Articles
Author, date, title of article, journal name, volume, number and pages.

Materials
Name of item, name and address of source, company, center or hospital, telephone number and approximate cost.

Group Session Outline
Session _____ of 6

A group session outline should be written for each of the six sessions of your group. Headings are as follows:
Group Title:
Session Title:
Format (time sequence):
Supplies:
Description:

Session _____ of 6

The session number (this session) of total number of sessions planned indicates sequence. Your group sessions should be planned in logical order, from simple to complex, superficial to deep, general to specific, etc. In a closed group the sessions should build on one another so that general group principles can be applied. It would make sense for the first session to be somewhat introductory, so that members begin to know not only the subject of the group, but each other as well. Subjects of a more personal nature should be saved for later in the sequence when members know one another better. The last session needs to deal with summary and termination of the group. The way you sequence the sessions will depend somewhat on your chosen population.

Group Title

This is the title of the group as a whole, for example, "Money Management."

Session Title

Like the group title, each session should be labeled with a word or phrase describing either the content or the goal for that session.

Format

This is a short outline stating what will happen when. For example, a session in "Balancing your Checkbook" might have the following format.
5 min - review last week
10 min - introductory lecturette
15 min - complete sample checkbook worksheet
10 min - check answers with calculator
20 min - discuss specific problems and summarize importance of balancing checkbook.
60 min - total
You need not include this last total figure, but make sure your timing fits the total time allotted for the group.

Supplies

This category includes a complete list of what is needed to complete the group. Do not assume patients will be carrying pens and pencils with them or will be wearing a watch. The supply list should include the correct number of each item needed. For a "Balancing Your Checkbook" session, supplies for a group of five patients would include the following:

5 worksheets (attach copy)
5 pencils
5 pocket calculators
1 large pad and 1 marker (for therapist to illustrate process)

Description

This is a step-by-step description of what will be included. The introduction should be fully described, including warm-up (if appropriate), explanation of purpose, expectations and time frame. If there are lecturettes, these must be outlined. If worksheets are to be written, a copy must be attached. Activities must be fully described including directions, choices, timing. If the activity was selected from a text or prior experience, reference should be given. For the discussion part, a list of questions to be asked is included. The discussion questions should be divided into the following categories: processing, generalizing and application. Refer to Chapter 1 for a description of these phases of the group. Your discussions will vary depending on the frame of reference you are using. It is wise to be prepared with more questions than you will need. Also keep in mind the goals of the group when choosing discussion questions. An activity is generally more effective when the patients feel it has meaning for them. Relating each session's activity back to the original goals will help keep both patients and therapist on track. A verbal summary at the end of each session is important. Include for each session some points to remember for the summary.

Instructions for Preparing Protocol

When you have written the entire protocol you should type it onto a word processor. Each session should start a new page. When putting on the word processor, use the exact headings in the order described. Capitalize the headings; use single spacing and 1" margins. It is not necessary to indent. Skip a line between each section or heading.

When rating sheets or worksheets are used, a copy should be attached to the outline or session to which it relates. Use the following forms to write your first draft of your Group Treatment Plan Protocol.

Group Treatment Plan Outline

Group Title:

Author:

Frame of Reference:

Purpose:

Group Membership and Size:

Group Goals:

1.

2.

3.

4.

5.

6.

7.

8.

Rationale:

Outcome Criteria:

Method:

Time and Place of Meeting:

Supplies and Cost:

References:

Group Title:

Session Title:

Format:

Supplies:

Description:

Group Title:

Session Title:

Format:

Supplies:

Description:

Group Title:

Session Title:

Format:

Supplies:

Description:

Group Title:

Session Title:

Format:

Supplies:

Description:

Group Title:

Session Title:

Format:

Supplies:

Description:

Group Title:

Session Title:

Format:

Supplies:

Description:

Note: James P. Klyczek is co-author of Chapter 10. Dr. Klyczek originated the concept of the group treatment plan assignment with the six session outlines in 1985, and very kindly shared his group dynamics course materials with me several years ago. Dr. Klyczek is Assistant Professor and Clinical Coordinator in the Occupational Therapy Program, Division of Health and Human Services, D'Youville College, Buffalo, New York.

Bibliography

American Psychological Association. Publication Manual. 3rd ed. Washington DC: APA, 1983.
AOTA. Uniform terminology for occupational therapy. 2nd ed. *AJOT*, 1989, 43, 12, 808-815.
Dunn W. and McGourty L. Application of uniform terminology to practice. *AJOT*, 1989, 43, 12, 817-831.

Chapter

11

A Group
Laboratory Experience

The following is an example of a group protocol. It is a group designed as a laboratory experience for professional students. Ideally it is done in groups of eight students, with the instructor as leader. It addresses some of the most common professional issues for students and serves as a context for the discussion of the principles of group dynamics described in Chapter 2. The series of six sessions is planned in a sequence that moves toward greater intimacy as the group develops. The leadership is also intended to change from directive in the beginning toward a democratic, facilitative style at the end. The group leader models therapeutic interventions with various problem behaviors and fosters the exploration of here and now relationships. Members have the opportunity to take on various roles and to practice group interaction skills. Process illumination should be discussed as a part of each session, with a goal of learning and personal growth. Although this is a six session sequence, it has been suggested by my students that three open sessions be interspersed.

An open session has no planned activity, and its purpose is to discuss the process of prior sessions. After session three in my group, for example, there seemed to be little time to discuss the many issues and feelings resulting from giving and receiving feedback. An open group following this session would give the members a chance to discuss their concerns and to better understand their relationship to each other. Session four seemed to be too structured, and several of the groups felt the need to voice their urge to rebel against the structure and/or the directive leadership style. An open session following this one would allow for the discussion of group development, and the significance of their rebellion in the context of group development theories. Another interesting addition to the sequence is a leaderless group. This forces the group members to take on leadership roles, and further illuminates the group process. This semester, many of the groups decided to end their group with a "termination" activity. One group brought in brunch, another had a pizza party and another decided on a good-bye collage. With these additions, the group lab experience is expanded to ten weekly sessions.

Group Treatment Plan Outline

Group Title: Developing Your Professional Self

Author: Marilyn B. Cole, MS, OTR

Frame of Reference: The frame of reference for this group is existential-humanistic. The assumption is that members are motivated to know themselves better and to become competent professionals.

Purpose: This group is designed to help junior occupational therapy students to make the transition from a student role to a professional role. The six group activities are selected to deal with the most common areas of difficulty for students, such as being assertive, accepting feedback and setting priorities in their lives.

Group Membership and Size: "Developing Your Professional Self" is designed for second semester junior occupational therapy students. Most of these students are between 20 and 22 years of age, although several are adults coming back to school. The majority are women who have lived independent of their families for at least two years, although there are several men and several students who commute from home. Having entered the junior year in an occupational therapy academic program, these students have all achieved and maintained a high academic average, and have survived at least one semester of difficult and challenging professional course work. All have had at least one semester of clinical Fieldwork I experiences, allowing them a taste of what it is like to work with patients (a few hours per week). In choosing to become occupational therapists, these students have set a goal and are working to achieve it.

This will be a closed group of no more than eight members. The same members will be expected to attend all six sessions with no absences.

Group Goals and Rationale: The student will:
1. Discuss awareness of professional self in relation to clients and peers.
2. Demonstrate ability to problem-solve, behave assertively and set goals and priorities.
3. Identify strengths and weaknesses of self and others.
4. Accept feedback from others and use it constructively.
5. Clearly state professional values.
6. Demonstrate ability to interact effectively with peers.
7. Identify group behaviors and group process.

Students in the junior year are learning many of the skills necessary to treat patients. However, in order to use those skills effectively, the student needs to feel comfortable in the professional role. The "Developing Your Professional Self" group is designed to promote a needed self-awareness associated with professionalism. As a professional team member, future occupational therapists will need to interact effectively, behave assertively when necessary, share in group problem solving, and learn constructively from other team members. Factors other than academic ones will influence professional effectiveness, such as warmth and empathy, flexibility and openness, ability to express feelings and appropriate self-disclosure. The group format gives students an opportunity to explore and practice needed skills and attributes in preparation for their Fieldwork II experiences.

This group design, although planned for occupational therapy students, may also be useful for students in other disciplines. Adaptations would be minimal, simply substituting for "occupational therapy," "nursing, physical therapy, social work" etc. The group and interpersonal skills needed by many health professionals are quite similar.

Outcome Criteria:
1. The student will demonstrate interpersonal skills by verbal participation at least three times in each weekly session.
2. Students within the context of each session will discuss and demonstrate the skills required for self-disclosure, problem-solving, giving and receiving feedback, empathizing with or confronting others, behaving assertively and setting goals and priorities.
3. The progress of each student may be rated twice on a 5 point scale, 1 being poor ability and 5 being excellent ability. The first rating should be before the first session, the second rating after the sixth session. This pre and post-group rating will then show progress made by each student in each skill required. The Group Member Progress Rating chart may be used to measure progress in each of these factors: self-disclosure, problem-solving, giving feedback, receiving feedback, empathizing with others, confronting others, behaving assertively, setting personal goals and understanding dynamics.

Group Member Progress Rating

Rating 1 (low) to 5 (high)	Session 1	Session 6
Self-disclosure	_____	_____
Problem-solving	_____	_____
Giving feedback	_____	_____
Receiving feedback	_____	_____
Empathizing with others	_____	_____
Confronting others	_____	_____
Behaving assertively	_____	_____
Setting goals	_____	_____
Understanding dynamics	_____	_____

Method:
Structured group activities and discussions will occur each week. The activities will be graded from a superficial and safe level to a deeper level interpersonally. The activities will also be graded so as to encourage more group interaction and less dependence on the leader as each week progresses. Group development and interpersonal learning will be encouraged, and an understanding of the process of the group will be facilitated.

Time and place of meeting:
The group will meet for one hour each week for six weeks. The rooms are selected to be free of noise distraction and to preserve the confidentiality of the group. A large table and nine chairs are preferable, so that members can work on group projects. On days when only discussion takes place, chairs may be arranged in a circle without the table. For the one hour meeting, it is important that no one leaves or comes late, and that there are no interruptions. The door should be closed, and a sign saying "Do Not Disturb, Group in Session" should be displayed outside.

Supplies and cost:

	unit price	total
9 sheets of white drawing paper 12"x18" - donated		
16 assorted magazines - donated		
5 jars of glue	$1.50	7.50
9 pair scissors	$2.50	22.50
10 marking pens (set)	$2.50	2.50
10 pencils (pack)	$1.50	1.50
1 package 3x5 index cards	$1.25	1.25
Xerox copies	.10	2.00
9 sheets typing paper - donated		
	Total cost	$37.25

Reference
Rider B. and Gramblin C. *Activities Card File*, 1987.

Group Session Outline
Session 1 of 6

Group Title: Developing Your Professional Self

Session Title: *Professional Self-Awareness Collage*
(adapted from Rider & Gramblin 1987)

Format:
Warm-up - 5 min.
Introduce group lab - 5 min.
Instructions for activity - 5 min.
Collage activity - 20 min.
Sharing - 15 min.
Discussion - 20 min.
Summary - 5 min.

Supplies:
9 sheets white drawing paper 12"x18"
5 jars of glue
9 pairs of scissors
16 uncut magazines
10 marking pens, assorted colors

Description:
1. Warm-up - Ask each person in turn to give his or her name and something he or she likes and doesn't like about occupational therapy.

2. Introduce activity (group lab) - Group Outline will be shared with the group.

3. Instructions for activity - The purpose of this activity is to help us think about ourselves as professionals. (Give out bags and markers) "We will begin by signing our name at the top like this 'Jane Doe, OTS.' (Magazines, glue and scissors are placed in center of table.) Look through the magazines and cut out pictures that represent qualities you have as a professional. We all have some characteristics that we will want to share and have others know about. These may be characteristics that will help us as a professional. Fold the drawing paper in half and paste the pictures representing these on the outside of the folder you have made. You may use both front and back covers. We also have some characteristics we would rather not share. These may be a hindrance to our professional identity. Cut out pictures representing these and paste them on the inside of the folder you have made. When you are finished pasting the pictures, use markers to label each with the characteristic you intend it to represent. You have about 20 minutes to complete this task. We will discuss the collages when we are finished. This will be a good way to get to know each other better." Give warning when 5 minutes are left. After 5 minutes, collect all materials and place out of reach.

4. Sharing - Ask for a volunteer to start sharing the collages. Once started, go around the group in order, forcing no one to share more than he or she wants.

5. Discussion questions -
Processing:
How did you feel about doing this?
How many of us felt comfortable sharing the outside vs inside of the folder?

Group Session Outline
Session 1 of 6 (continued)

Generalizing:
How well do you know your professional self?
What did you learn about yourself from doing this activity?
What did you learn about others?
How difficult was it to decide which parts of yourself are "professional?"

Application:
How will an activity like this help people build a professional identity?

6. Summary - Points to remember are to be taken from comments of members. Some might be:
a) the "face" we show to the public is not what's really inside.
b) The outside represents what we wish to be, the inside what we fear we may be.
c) Students do not find it easy to think of themselves as professional.
d) Some common characteristics are the wish to play a helping role and fondness and empathy for other people.

Group Session Outline
Session 2 of 6

Group Title: Developing Your Professional Self

Session Title: *Difficult Decisions*

Format:
Warm-up - 5 min.
Introduce activity - 5 min.
Instructions for activity - 5 min.
Difficult decision writing - 10 min.
Discussion - 35 min.
Summary - 5 min.

Supplies:
8 3x5 index cards
8 pencils
Basket or box ("hat")

Description:
1. Warm-up - ask members to give names and recall one characteristic about their professional self from last session.

2. Introduce activity - "Today we will discuss difficult professional decisions or problems. Each of you take an index card and a pencil and write on the card a professional problem or decision you have experienced in the last year. You may draw on Fieldwork I experiences, volunteer experiences or situations in the classroom, as long as they concern some aspect of your chosen profession."

3. Instructions for activity - "You can write about a problem you had difficulty with or had trouble making a decision about. Give necessary background and detail, but you need not identify yourself. We will be putting the cards in a hat and drawing out someone else's problem to solve. You have 10 minutes to write your problem." Give 1 minute warning.

   Collect all cards after 10 minutes and shuffle them - put back in "hat" and ask each member to draw one out. If someone draws his own, he has the option of putting it back and drawing another. "Now think about the problem on the card you drew and get ready to share with the group how you would solve it. Take turns sharing solutions and discuss."

   For this activity, discussion will be during the sharing rather than afterward. Members have the option of identifying their problem and asking the group for additional help.

4. Discussion questions -
   Processing:
   What feelings are involved?
   How does it feel to need/ask for help?

Generalizing:
   Whose problem is it? Should it be?
   What did you/others contribute?
   What is the worst/best thing you could do?
   If decision, what are pros and cons?
   Whose decision is it?
   Should it be?
   What additional info is needed to decide/solve?

Application:
   What can we learn from each other as professionals?
   How can we help each other as professionals?

5. Summary - This activity usually produces much discussion and often members own up to their own problem. They have become a group of peers working together, and trusting one another. A parallel should be drawn to the ideal in practice where no one should feel afraid to ask the help of their colleagues in facing a difficult problem.

Group Session Outline
Session 3 of 6

Group Title: Developing Your Professional Self

Session Title: *Giving and Receiving Feedback*

Format:
Warm-up - 5 min.
Introduce activity - 5 min.
Instructions for activity - 5 min.
Writing activity - 15 min.
Discussion - 20 min.
Summary - 5 min.

Supplies:
9 sheets of paper 8-1/2 x 11
9 pens or pencils

Description:
1. Warm-up - Begin by asking members to say a few words about how they are feeling today.

2. Introduce activity - "Today we will be working on communication, self-awareness and accepting feedback from others. Often the success of our professional interactions will depend on how well we understand our own feelings and express them to others. Even negative feelings can be expressed in positive terms. For example, if you are studying for a test, and your roommate is talking loudly on the phone, you might say to her 'I know you're enjoying talking to your friend, but I'm having a hard time concentrating on my work. Would you mind calling your friend back later?' "

   "Most people have an easier time giving positive feedback than negative. However, avoiding negative comments can cause all kinds of problems, especially when two people have to work together. This exercise is designed to practice giving positive and negative feedback to each other."

3. Instructions for activity - Pass out paper and pencils. Instructions are: "Fold paper in half. Put name on the outside folded half at the top. On the inside, write some ways you feel *you* need to grow professionally (skills needed, issues to deal with, etc.). Fold paper over so what you have written is not visible. Pass folded paper around circle - each person writes on the *outside* how he feels the person whose name is on the paper could grow professionally. To make this chore less difficult, you may also write one thing you admire about the person. Both positive and 'change needed' comments should be expressed constructively. Even if you don't know everyone that well, do the best you can."

   Give 15 minutes for this part - after that stop, even if not finished. Each reads own paper for a few minutes. Then members share the result with the group. If possible, each should read a few positive and growth comments to the group.

Group Session Outline
Session 3 of 6 (continued)

4. Discussion questions -

Processing:

How do you feel about the feedback you received?

How did you feel about giving feedback to others?

What problems did you encounter in doing this exercise?

Generalizing:

How do the comments about yourself compare with comments of others?

What feedback from others do you agree/disagree with?

What did you learn from doing this exercise?

Application:

Whom would you like feedback from in your professional role?

How can you use feedback in everyday life?

How can you become more comfortable in giving constructive feedback to others? To patients?

5. Summary - Ask members to summarize.

Group Session Outline
Session 4 of 6

Group Title: Developing Your Professional Self

Session Title: *Professional Values*

Format:
Warm-up - 5 min.
Introduce activity - 5 min.
Instructions for activity - 5 min.
Activity - 15 min.
Discussion - 35 min.
Summary - 5 min.

Supplies:
9 pencils
9 values work sheets

Description:
1. Warm-up - Begin by summarizing last week's activity. How are people left feeling about the group? Is there any unfinished business? (Any comments, either negative or positive, should be accepted by the leader without judgment and acknowledged.

2. Introduce activity - "Knowing our professional values can help us set priorities and use our time at work and away from work more constructively. For example: If I want to balance my career with a meaningful relationship with my family, then I will be careful not to work overtime or make work-related commitments on weekends. Professional values should also guide our behavior at work. If you believe a good rapport with patients is important, you may take extra time with them to show your concern."
   Pass out values worksheets and pencils. Follow instructions on top of sheet. Allow 15 minutes to complete. When finished, each member shares his responses with the group.

3. Instructions for activity - The discussion guidelines written on the sheet are to come up with a group consensus on values held in common.

   (Generalizing is done by the group.)

   One group member can be a recorder and allow group to collaborate on what professional values they can agree on. A separate values worksheet may be used for note taking of group values.

4. Discussion questions -
   Processing:
   How members felt about doing the activity should be discussed.

   Application:
   What role do values play in your professional life?
   How do values determine how you spend your time?

5. Summary - In summary, the recorder can read her notes back to the group and accept final revisions and/or comments.

Values Worksheet

Instructions: Complete the following sentences in your own words. Then compare your responses to those of the other members of your group in order to generate a set of commonly held values in interpersonal relations. In the discussion, you have four tasks: 1) to make yourself heard, 2) to hear others accurately, 3) to listen for themes and 4) to collaborate on the group consensus.

A professional should:

A professional should not:

A supervisor:

A student:

A colleague:

A spouse or boyfriend/girlfriend:

I want to be remembered as a person who:

Our group:

Group Session Outline
Session 5 of 6

Group Title: Developing Your Professional Self

Session Title: *Assertiveness Role Play*

Format:
Warm-up - 5 min.
Introduce activity - 5 min.
Instructions for activity - 5 min.
Activity writing - 15 min.
Sharing (role playing)- 30 min.
Discussion - 10 min.
Summary - 10 min.

Supplies:
8 Index cards, 8 pencils

Description:
1. Warm-up - define assertive, passive and aggressive and discuss the differences between these.
2. Introduce activity - "One of the most common problems students have in making the transition to professionals is not acting assertively. Lack of assertiveness can lead to difficulty even on fieldwork experiences, as many of you have already discovered. For example, one student on a Fieldwork I experience overheard a discussion by staff members who were setting up a family conference in the patient lounge at 2 o'clock. This student was already scheduled to run an occupational therapy group in that room at 2 o'clock. However, she did not say anything about it to the staff group. The student was left without a place to run group and became very frustrated. Afterward, when staff became aware of the problem, they wondered why the student didn't speak up! They could have met in several other places. This situation could have been avoided if the student had behaved more assertively."
3. Instructions for activity - pass out index cards and pencils. "You will now write down on the card a professional situation in which would like to have responded more assertively but did not. You may either have been too passive or overly aggressive instead. On the front of the card, describe the situation; who, what, where and when, and whatever background information is necessary. On the back, state what your actual response was (if possible give a quote) and state how you felt afterward."
4. Sharing - each member shares the situation written on the front of the card. Then members decide as a group which situations they would like to role play. Group chooses a first, second and third choice, using group decision-making techniques to do this.

   Role play one to three situations as time allows:
   a) allow protagonist to direct role play
   b) protagonist chooses members of group to play significant characters
   c) protagonist sets up room, props
   d) role play situation as it really happened first, then discuss
   e) reverse roles and play situation using assertive behavior as discussed by the group
   f) allow a few alter egos to present feelings, and/or alternate responses

Group Session Outline
Session 5 of 6 (continued)

4. Discussion questions -

Processing:

How did you feel about doing the role play?

Which characters did you identify with?

How do you feel about being assertive? passive? aggressive?

What are you feeling about the protagonist's situation?

Generalizing:

What passive, assertive and aggressive behaviors can you identify in the role play?

What are the advantages of assertive behavior?

Application:

What did you learn about being assertive professionally?

What steps do you personally need to take to be able to behave assertively in the professional setting? As a student? As an occupational therapist?

5. Summary - Summarize by reinforcing assertive behaviors, reviewing the role of feelings and habits and thanking role players for their participation.

Group Session Outline
Session 6 of 6

Group Title: Developing Your Professional Self

Session Title: *Group Evaluation*

Format:
    Warm-up - 5 min.
    Introduce activity - 5 min.
    Instructions for activity - 5 min.
    Activity - 15 min.
    Discussion - 20 min.
    Summary of all six sessions - 15 min.

Supplies:
    9 Group Evaluation sheets
    9 Pencils

Description:

1. Warm-up - Begin by stating that this will be the final group of the series and ask members to say how they feel about ending the group.

2. Introduce activity - "An important part of the termination of groups is to review all the sessions and summarize what has been valuable. As professionals, we will all need to evaluate our patient groups, so this will be good practice. The Group Evaluation Worksheet has been designed to help you think specifically about this group and to apply some of what you have learned about group dynamics. (Give out worksheets). First, you are asked to identify the roles your fellow members played in the groups, and for this you will have to name names. In our discussion, these questions will serve as the basis of giving one another feedback about our participation. Next, we will look at the events of the group. These are emotionally charged situations which often emerge unexpectedly. In the context of activities, often it is the conflicts and problems groups encounter which become the turning points from which we learn the most. You are asked to identify three such events over the last five sessions.

    Norms are the "ground rules" of behavior in groups. You are asked to identify the implicit or implied norms over the course of the group. The stage of development is sometimes difficult to identify in the short time this group has been meeting. We will use Schutz's stages of inclusion, control and affection as a guide (Chapter 2). Sometimes the characteristics of stages overlap and this can be confusing, so you are asked to justify your choice with behaviors you see/have seen in this group. Your feeling about the group may be an important clue about what stage the group has achieved. Finally, you are asked to look at the group leadership. What style was used, and how has it changed over the course of the group? You have 15 minutes to complete the worksheet."

3. Instructions for activity - Members share their answers to some, or all of the questions on the sheet, as time allows. After each question, ask the group to discuss their answers and come to a consensus. Be sure to leave the last 15 minutes to summarize.

Group Session Outline
Session 6 of 6 (continued)

4. Discussion questions -
   Summary of all six sessions - Take a few minutes to reflect on the past six sessions.
   Processing:
   > What parts of the group experience are most memorable?
   > Which experiences did you like best/least?
   > How do you feel about your role in the group?

   Generalizing:
   > What things did you learn from being a part of this group?

   Application:
   > What parts of this group experience can you take with you and apply to future roles both personally and professionally?

5. Summary - End by summarizing results and asking each person to say in their own words, what parts of this group experience they value and feel good about.

Group Evaluation Worksheet

Directions: Answer the following questions about your group as it has developed from Session 1. Be sure to identify members by name.

Participation and Roles:
1. Who are the most outspoken participants?

2. Who are the least frequent participants?

3. Who talks to whom? What patterns have you observed? (Identify any sub-groups that exist)

4. Who keeps the ball rolling?

5. Who/what has blocked the group?

6. What rivalries have you observed during the group? Who has challenged the leadership?

Events: Name three interactions or situations which were high points or turning points for the group. Describe each situation briefly.

1.

2.

3.

Norms:
1. What behaviors are acceptable to the group today?

2. What behaviors are not acceptable today?

3. How have norms changed from the beginning of the group?

Stage of Development:
1. What stage of development has this group achieved? Justify your answer.
   a. Inclusion
   b. Control
   c. Affection

2. How do you feel about the group right now?
   a. It means a lot to me. I'm sorry it's ending.
   b. I feel good about the other members.
   c. I feel indifferent.
   d. It feels uncomfortable. I'm glad it's ending.
   e. I strongly dislike the group.

Leadership:
1. What was the leader's style of leadership? Why?
   a. Directive
   b. Facilitator
   c. Leader as adviser

2. How has the role of the leader changed over the course of the group?

Contract for Group Membership

This contract should be reviewed and signed by each member of the group before beginning the first session.

I understand I am involved in a developmental process and therefore it's necessary to attend all sessions to benefit fully from the process.

I realize that in order for me to be an effective member, it is important that I complete all assignments and arrive on time.

I agree to participate as openly, honestly and responsibly as I am able to, realizing that I am not under any group pressure to reveal personal data that I would regret sharing with the group.

I agree to speak personally and make "I" statements as objectively and specifically as I can, trying not to generalize or talk in abstractions.

I realize that no personal information about any group member should ever be discussed outside of the group.

Signed _____ Date _____

Appendices

A - The Task-Oriented Group as a Context
for Treatment

B - The Concept and Use of Developmental
Groups

C - Summary of Mosey's Adaptive Skills

D - Uniform Terminology for Occupational
Therapy—Third Edition

E - Comparison of Group Leadership
Guidelines in Seven Frames of Reference

Appendix
A

The Task-Oriented Group As A Context for Treatment*

Gail S. Fidler, OTR

Abstract

Increasing recognition of the influence of man's social and cultural environment on behavior has extended the parameters of patient treatment. Such developments are manifested in the gradual melding of sociologic, psychoanalytic and learning theories and the emerging focus on ego functions and adaptive skills. This paper explores concepts of the task-oriented group within this context, offering a definition and delineation of purpose for its use in occupational therapy as a remedial-learning experience for the schizophrenic patient.

Returning the hospitalized psychiatric patient to an acceptable productive role in the community and appreciably reducing the rate of recidivism is a complex problem. Such concern has led to intensive studies of both psychotherapeutic procedures and organizational structures of the mental hospital. The impact of sociologic inquiry into the mental hospital has been to add another dimension to our theoretical constructs regarding both individual feeling and behavior, and conditions under which such behavior may be altered to the benefit of the patient.

Understanding the significance of the social matrix in which the patient functions has brought more sharply into focus factors influencing ego function in addition to the intrapsychic and intrapersonal. As early as 1931 Harry Stack Sullivan[1] spoke of the importance of the social setting to the behavior of schizophrenic patients. Literature of the past fifteen years is replete with the investigations and analyses of the import of environment on patient functioning.[2-4] This focus has inevitably led to theoretical and practical attempts to relate concepts of ego psychology to social theories of the environment.[5-6] Such linkage as well as the social scientist's interest in group phenomena has given impetus to increased exploration of the many facets of group process and group therapy.

©AJOT XXIII, 1, 1969. Reprinted with permission.

Group Process and Group Psychotherapy

Group psychotherapy is firmly established as a method of treatment for mental illness. It has its foundation in psychodynamic personality theories and emerged in America essentially from a psychoanalytic frame of reference stressing personality change through exploration of intrapsychic and interpersonal pathology believed to be at the root of conflicts and problems.[7-10] The group has been seen as a setting in which the individual with the help of the therapist and through sharing with other members could explore and work through those unconscious conflicts and problems which inhibited personality change and growth. Such a frame of reference places primary importance on unconscious phenomena and explores here-and-now feelings and behavior as a means to arriving at an awareness and understanding of intrapsychic conflict. The role of the therapist is to facilitate such awareness and elicit the involvement and help of members in exposing and working through personal conflicts and problems.

The social scientist's interest in groups emanated from a sociologic orientation rather than from personality theories. This frame of reference stresses the impact of society and the group on individual behavior and seeks to explain behavior based on the nature of the society in which a man lives. This ideology is exemplified by Lewin[11] who theorized that behavior was determined by the situation in which it occurred as well as by personality factors. The sociologist's beginning involvement with groups was via his interest in organizational structure and this was reflected in an early focus on the use of the group to accomplish a task or to effect a change in management.[12] Such experimentation inevitably led to the development of theories regarding the use of such groups in teaching and learning.[13]

Theories and practice in the field of group dynamics have focused on the group as a dynamic force in facilitating learning and behavioral change. Emphasis on "the group" as the primary change-producing agent thus accentuates the importance of exploring the dynamic forces within the here-and-now group to both understand and facilitate such change. Group structure and membership roles become significant and individual feeling and behavior is viewed only as it contributes to or deters from cohesive structure and contributory roles.

As the group therapist, the psychiatrist and social scientist work collaboratively in an attempt to resolve some of the complex problems of the mentally ill, these two seemingly disparate theories have moved closer together. There are increasing efforts to integrate not only practice of group psychotherapy and group dynamics but also the more apparently divergent concepts of each. One has but to survey current literature to be impressed with the ubiquity of these efforts.

Experimental Studies

In "Social Psychology In Treating Mental Illness"[14] Fairweather describes an experimental approach combining the psychodynamic doctrine of patient treatment with theories of social psychiatry, sociology and the small group. This program focused around patient-led, small task-oriented groups for the chronic regressed schizophrenic. Such an approach, Dr. Fairweather points out, "called for an altered perception of the patient's role from that of a subordinate to that of a peer group member with responsiblities to himself and his group members, and away from that of a passive recipient within the limits of his abilities, despite existing psychopathology."[15] Tasks around which these autonomous patient-led groups were organized concerned the current and future living of each member. Thus task levels ranged according to the capacity of the patient from personal care and ward responsibility to responsiblity for vocational planning and placement. These groups provided the opportunity for patients to explore and develop their capacities for independent function, creating patient roles within the hospital which were more consistent with those of the outside community.

This study made an important contribution to patient programming and treatment. Although it concerned itself entirely with problems of the chronic regressed schizophrenic, there is much that would seem to be directly applicable to other patient catagories and most certainly to patient groups in rehabilitation settings.

Marshall Edelson's experimental study[6] at the University of Oklahoma was concerned with "making possible the meaningful integration of both group experience and individual psychotherapy in an intensive treatment program designed to accomplish fundamental alteration in characterological disorder rather than solely rapid relief of acute secondary symptomatology and restoration of an ability to function marginally in the community." This work combines ego psychology and group dynamics in a therapeutic community as the basis for intensive psychotherapy. The focus of this study is aptly stated by Dr. Edelson in these words: "The therapeutic community (and small group) is organized to provide opportunities for the appearance of the patient's characterological difficulties or way of life as these are expressed in activities and other aspects of group living and for the confrontation of the patient and the group with these difficulties and their consequences to the life of the (hospital) community."

A third innovative experiment was Robert Morton's use of the laboratory method with psychiatric patients.[17] This study describes the design and use of the group process laboratory training program for hospitalized mental patients. The laboratory is a structured, small group experience designed to bring about change by establishing conditions whereby participants are forced to test their assumptions regarding interpersonal and group relations. Not only is the application of the laboratory experience to hospitalized psychiatric patients a creative innovation, but it is even more provocative to learn that they were autonomous, staff-leaderless, patient groups. Morton agrees with Fairweather that cohesive decision-making groups with psychotics cannot be explored if a professional leader is present. It is their contention that even the most permissive therapist-leader reinforces dependency for the psychotic to a detrimental extent. This experiment provides some useful and creative postulates regarding small group experiences for psychiatric patients and should stimulate further research and study in the adaptation of this technique in treatment and rehabilitation programs.

It is interesting to note that in follow-up studies on the Morton experiment only two findings seemed to be suggestive.[18] Training laboratory patients were employed a mean of 5.92 months during the nine month follow-up period whereas the group therapy patients were employed 4.70 months. In the Fairweather study, patients participating in the small-group program were significantly better than the control group in community adjustment with regard to areas of employment, verbal communication with others and friendships.

These three experimental studies are examples of the way in which the small group is being used and adapted to meet treatment needs and essentially bridge the apparent gap between theories of individual psychodynamics and sociology.

The Task Group in Occupational Therapy

Development of task-oriented treatment groups approximately four years ago within the occupational therapy program at New York State Psychiatric Institute emanated from several not unrelated observations. First, the increasing conviction that as patients engaged in activities or created objects they expressed characterological difficulties and that attention to these problems as they emerged and were operant in the here and now seemed to be of benefit to the patient. Second, a seemingly evident relationship between problems evidenced by the patient in his activity experiences and difficulties he encountered in the work-day world. Third, the nature of the occupational therapy setting which expects active involvement in doing, provides a microcosm of life-work situations which can be seen and explored as they occur rather than in retrospect. Fourth, recognition of the relationships between verbal skills and learning and our experience which indicated that learning and concomitant growth were enhanced when problems in doing were identified and explored. Finally, our belief that the shared, small group experience is conducive to the exploration and amelioration of some problems in ego function.

Groups were organized with approximately eight members selected on the basis of their particular difficulties in doing and being productive as well as their readiness and need for a small group experience. All patients admitted to these early groups were male schizophrenics and placement in a given group was determined by the level of ego function. Meetings were held three to four times a week for periods of one and one-half hours. Each group was responsible for choosing its own common task and arriving at a consensus regarding procedures for accomplishing that task.

Definition and Purpose

Task as it relates to such groups is defined as any activity or process directed toward creating or producing an end product or demonstrable service for the group as a whole and/or for persons outside of the group. Some examples of tasks chosen by these groups were: publishing a newspaper, cooking, building a playhouse for the childrens' service, gardening, organizing a patient council, play reading and ward decoration and improvement.

The intent of the task-oriented group is to provide a shared working experience wherein the relationship between feeling, thinking and behavior, their impact on others and on task accomplishment and productivity can be viewed and explored. Alternate patterns of functioning can be considered and tested within the context of the here and now, to the end that such learning may induce ego growth and improve function. Task accomplishment is not the purpose of the group but hopefully the means by which purpose is realized. It is seen as the catalytic agent which elicits behavior and interaction, brings into focus both functional capacities and limitations, facilitates collaboration in working through problems and provides a concrete reality factor against which to measure learning and achievement. Furthermore, the task provides a frame of reference which helps to keep in focus what is relevant to explore and work through and what conflicts and issues belong more appropriately in other treatment settings. In such a group, issues and problems which directly effect the cohesiveness and/or task accomplishment are the appropriate agenda items.

Such groups are not unique in eliciting or diagnosing conflicts of the schizophrenic but it would seem that use of a common task within a small group setting does facilitate delineation of certain problems and their amelioration. Responsibility for selecting and accomplishing a task provides an opportunity for the group to explore problem-solving and decision-making skills, to have concrete evidence of their ability to function as well as to identify those expectations which give rise to conflict. The expectation that an activity needs to be chosen and implemented makes it necessary for the group to look at concepts regarding self and others that have impaired problem-solving skills and gives impetus to working toward their resolution.

The ability to perceive cause and effect relationships is a well-recognized problem of the schizophrenic and learning in this area requires consistent, repeated opportunities to see and have evidence of cause and effect. The task-oriented group with its focus on the relationship between feelings, thinking, behavior and task achievement thus creates excellent learning opportunities. Following through on a task procedure, the nature of doing or not doing, gives ample confirmation of cause and effect regarding behavior and function. When task responsibility must be shared and when the nature of one's doing is viewed in terms of its contribution to the group, such learning is further amplified.

Reality testing through consensual validation is an essential process in every group and is of particular value to the schizophrenic. In addition to the shared reality indigenous to group structure and interaction, a clearly delineated task with standard procedures and techniques provides a shared reality from which perceptions can be tested and shared. Shared participation in an activity, the necessary interdependence makes possible an objective, demonstrable assessment of one's capacities and limitations. One of the values of the task-oriented group is the consensual validation of the patients' capacity to grow and change as evidenced in the accomplishment of a task.

The need to work together as well as talk together about one's doing contributes to learning to conceptualize and verbalize more accurately and directly. Identification of problems in functioning, discussion of these as well as exploration of alternatives, combines feeling, behavior and cognition and provides the necessary components of learning and change. The shared decision-making, working experiences available in these groups and the opportunity to explore and work through problems that interfere with satisfactory function make integrated learning possible. If we are to teach new and better ways of functioning then we need to combine the patient's doing with his thinking and bring such relationships into awareness in order that he may integrate such learning.

Collaboration on a concrete, clearly defined task encourages more direct and clear communication and coupled with group support provides a safe area in which to practice such skills. In addition, experiences in working and sharing help the schizophrenic to begin to perceive and conceptualize his needs within the context of gratification potential with increasing awareness of his own potential for obtaining gratification rather that the expectation of rejection or frustration outside himself.

The task-oriented group with its focus on function related to here-and-now tasks and doing their corresponding responsibilities bear a closer resemblance to living in the outside community and provides learning which correlates more directly with those skills and expectations required in community adjustment.

It would seem useful at this time to make some distinction between these groups and verbal psychotherapy and delineate some values to the patient when both experiences are correlated. Within the task-oriented group setting, issues concerning feelings, perceptions and behavior are discussed and explored only insofar as they are shared by others and impede or contribute to the problem-solving and/or activity accomplishment of the group. Personal, intrapsychic and historical determinants are not emphasized but are reserved for investigation in psychotherapy. Many personal and interpersonal percep-tions and responses are elicited but not dealt with in the group. Psychotherapy provides an opportunity to explore these in depth, interrelating the unconscious, the historical, the personal and interpersonal to the here and now. Likewise, the task-oriented group

275

provides a life-like action and doing setting in which insights gained in psychotherapy can be tested and consolidated through performance. The extent to which the task-oriented group and psychotherapy is correlated, the degree which the purpose of each and their relationship is understood by both staff and patients, may well determine the extent to which treatment potential will be realized.

Leadership

The role of staff leader or therapist is an important determinant in the group. The function of the leader is to facilitate a process and milieu which will be conducive to the kind of learning and growth to which these groups are directed. The role of the leader is to make learning possible and not to assume responsibility for the group. Fulfillment of objectives will depend in good measure on the leader's concepts of the mental patient and himself, as well as his skill in group and interpersonal processes.

Confidence in the inherent capacity of the group to be constructively self-determining, in its ability to ultimately recognize problems and reach realistic solutions to these, is a basic requirement. The foundation for such an attitude is belief in the right of the patient to be self-determining and a trust sufficient to allow exercise of freedom in exploring and testing his capacities. The group needs to be perceived as a therapeutic agent in its own right and leadership not as giving treatment but rather as the agent which helps to maximize the therapeutic and learning potential of the group.

It would seem that we tend to see patients as more fragile and thus needing more guidance and direction than seems warranted, at least on the basis of our experience. Perhaps this view of the patient is sustained by our need to be needed and important to the patient and to be recognized as having expertise. Autocratic leadership confirms for the patient his dependent position and tends to reaffirm his concept of self as inept and inadequate, while hesitant, aloof permissiveness increases his sense of vagueness, unpredictability and limitlessness. Jay W. Fidler[19] defines the nature and extent of leader activity as it pertains to working with groups of psychotics, emphasizing the importance of active interventions based on sensitivity and understanding of the schizophrenic's particular problems with reality testing and other ego functions.

Such understanding and attitude sets however, are not the only basis of leadership skills for these groups. An intimate knowledge of and skill in problem-solving procedures is essential if the group is to be helped toward learning and developing such capacities. The extent to which problem-solving skills are an inherent part of the leader's way of thinking and functioning and his ability to make these appropriately apparent in identifying and dealing with issues will, by and large, determine the extent to which the group will be able to learn these processes and incorporate them into their functioning.

The extent and quality of the leader's receptivity to looking at himself and his relations to others, his freedom to participate in the learning and growth process, his ability to share perceptions and his openness to exploring all aspects of his functioning in the group, will either make learning and growth possible and a less threatening expectation for members, or confirm the many doubts and distortions they bring to the experience. The leader cannot expect from his group what he is not willing or able to do himself.

Problems of the Schizophrenic

Several aspects of the task-oriented group seem to bring into focus particular problems of the schizophrenic patient. *First,* decision-making is particularly difficult, especially the decision regarding task choice. There seems to be little question that groups expect the staff leader to make the choice for them. Some groups have insisted that this be done while others have behaved as though this was what they both wanted and expected. Groups have discussed their anxieties and conflicts about decision-making and these discussions suggest that problems in this area are related to dependency needs, fear of responsibility and the ultimate unacceptability of any decision they might make. It would seem that since they conceptualize themselves as worthless and "bad", any decision they make as well as its implementation will be worthless and "bad" and reflect basic ineptness and inadequacy. It would also seem they expect authority (the parental figure) to find any decision they make unacceptable and inadequate. However, groups resent and may forcefully reject any task choice suggestion made by the leader. Ambivalence with regard to dependency, coupled with problems related to self-concept, compose one of the major conflictual areas which need to be worked through before meaningful growth can occur. Some of these findings would seem to support Fairweather's hypothesis that the dependency needs of the psychotic contraindicate staff leadership in task-oriented groups.

More recently we have been experimenting with a standard task for each beginning group in an effort to assess the extent to which decision-making problems may be altered or reduced when task choice is not an initial requirement. It is further hoped that such a procedure may lead to the development of a group diagnostic implement. However, the issue is not so much whether we deny or gratify the patient's dependency needs but rather how we can teach decision-making. It seems reasonable to conjecture that teaching such skills is a problem because of our limited understanding of the full nature of blocks to learning and thus our inability to identify and utilize techniques and procedures which facilitate learning.

Second, expectations of a shared group are frightening. It is as though fluid ego boundaries and difficulties in perceiving self as separate from others makes the closeness inherent in the small group an additional threat to identity. For some patients there is also the expectation that narcissistic needs will be frustrated and that sharing in a group will deny dependency needs. In addition, anticipation of shared doing seems to represent a threat to the schizophrenic's defenses and orientation. However, the structured, predictable aspects of the task and engagement with non-human objects increase opportunities for supportive consensual validation of observable abilities and facilitates identification of those perceptions which they share in common.

Third, great difficulty is experienced in problem-solving. Although some of the dilemmas operant in problem-solving are obviously related to dependency needs and authority relationships, difficulties which emerge in these groups suggest also that many patients have never learned even the basic procedures for identifying problems and exploring possible solutions, or have lost the ability to appropriately perceive and organize perceptions into logical concepts.

The combined thinking and doing, the cognitive perceptual skills at both the motor and verbal level inherent in the product of these groups, seem to bring clearly into focus disturbances and abilities in thinking and learning.

Fears associated with learning and related conflicts, disturbances in cognition and resultant dysfunction become readily evident. By the same token, the structure and focus of these groups make possible a sense of competence and learning less conflictual, the task providing evidence of movement toward achievement. Task activity furthermore creates opportunities to engage and relate in a more concrete way making it possible to be involved at a conceptual level commensurate with current capacities rather than consistently requiring a higher symbolic thinking order. The task also facilitates gradation of learning. As we become more knowledgeable about blocks to learning and their impact on function we should be able to articulate more meaningfully related learning experiences and use more fully the potential of the task-oriented group.

Finally, two generalized responses have been evident in these groups. There are those who find expectations of doing, the intrinsic action, learning and responsibilities, very threatening. These patients place a high premium on talking about their problems and intellectualization is used as a way of avoiding the more hazardous and fearful doing of a task. These groups have great difficulty arriving at a choice of task and such a decision may be prolonged for an inordinate period of time. Other patients seem driven to an excessive emphasis on the task, to a flight into activity as a means for avoiding bringing problems into awareness and working them through. Furthermore there would seem to be a correlation between the leader's characteristic way of functioning, what he perceives as the more important "therapeutic set" and a group's sustained focus or movement toward a more equitable balance between these two responses.

One further observation would seem to be useful and this relates to the kind of task choices made by groups. There seems to be an identifiable relationship between the task selected by a group, the level and nature of their primary emotional needs and the conflicts surrounding those needs. Furthermore, task choice seems to reflect the group's progress or regression. Further study of this phenomenon should increase our understanding of need-gratifying processes and enhance our ability to make growth potential opportunities available to the patients.

Returning the schizophrenic patient to the community as a potentially productive, contributing member with an increased capacity to sustain such a role, is a multi-faceted, complex problem. The task-oriented group represents one of many attempts to reduce the problem. It seems that at least it provides a structure wherein dysfunction can be observed and explored. Hopefully these and other explorations will make it possible to ultimately articulate more clearly the essential factors of remedial processes. As we become increasingly able to inter-relate psychodynamic and sociologic concepts, as we enhance our knowledge of the cognitive process and its relationships to intrapsychic phenomena and overt behavior, our efforts may come closer to realizing the ultimate goal of satisfactory community living for our patients.

Acknowledgement

The author is indebted to Dr. Lothar Gidro-Frank and Dr. Eugene Friedberg for their interested support and to Miss Patricia Mayer, OTR, whose creative thinking and skillful leadership contributed so much to our learning.

References

1. Sullivan, Harry Stack, "Socio-psychiatric Research: It's implications for The Scizophrenic Problem and Mental Hygiene", *Amer J Psychiat* Vol 10, 1931.
2. Stanton, AH and Schwartz, MS, *The Mental Hospital*, Basic Books, 1954.
3. Caudill, William, *The Psychiatric Hospital as a Small Society*, Harvard Univ. Press, 1958.
4. Jones, Maxwell, *The Therapeutic Community: A New Treatment Method in Psychiatry*, Basic Books, 1953.
5. Cummings, J and Cummings E, *Ego and and Milieu*, Atherton Press, NY, 1963.
6. Edelson, M, *Ego Psychology, Group Dynamics and the Therapeutic Community*, Grune & Stratton, NY, 1964.
7. Slavison, S, *Group Psychoanalytic Psychotherapy*, Interantional Univ. Press, NY, 1964.
8. Wolf, A, "The Psychoanalysis of Groups", *Amer J Psychother* Vol. 3, 1949.
9. Bach, G., *Intensive Group Psychotherapy*, The Ronald Press, NY, 1954.
10. Mullan, H and Rosenbaum, M, *Group Psychotherapy, Theory and Practice*, Glencoe Free Press, 1962.
11. Lewin, K, *Dynamic Theory of Personality*, McGraw Hill 1945.
12. Schien, E and Bennis, W, *Personal and Organizational Change Through Group Methods*, John Wiley & Sons, NY, 1965, 357-368.

13. Bradford, L., Gibb, J. and Benne, K., *T-Group Theory & Laboratory Method*, John Wiley & Sons, NY, 1964.

14. Fairweather, G.W., *Social Psychology in Treating Mental Illness*, John Wiley & Sons, NY, 1964.

15. Ibid. 14

16. Ibid. 6

17. Morton, R.B., "The Uses of the Laboratory Method in a Psychiatric Hospital", in *Personal and Organizational Change Through Group Methods*.

18. Johnson, D.L., Hanson, P.G., Rothaus, R., Morton, R.B., Lyle, E., and Moyer, R., "Follow up Evaluation of Human Relation Training for Psychiatric Patients", in *Personal and Organizational Change Through Group Methods*.

19. Fidler, J.W., "Group Psychotherapy of Psychotics", *Amer J Orthopsychiat* Vol. XXXV, No. 4, 1965.

Appendix

B

The Concept and Use of Developmental Groups

Anne Cronin Mosey, PhD, OTR

Developmental groups are task-oriented groups structured in such a manner as to stimulate the various types of nonfamilial groups usually encountered in the normal development process. Five types have been identified: parallel, project, egocentric-cooperative, cooperative, and mature. The concept of developmental groups was formulated in an attempt to apply recapitulation of ontogeny in the treatment of patients who are deficient in their ability to interact effectively in small groups. In dealing with this area of dysfunction, consecutive participation in the various types of developmental groups provides a framework for planned change. Group experiences are graded so as to provide opportunities for acquisition of basic group interaction skills. It is suggested that learning occurs through reinforcement of behaviors or approximation of behaviors that are necessary for successful participation in a given type of developmental group and nonreinforcement of behaviors that are inconsistent with successful participation.

A subtle change in orientation seems to be taking place among practitioners and scientists. There is movement away from the medical model, with its focus on concepts of pathology, toward an organization of thinking and effort around the concepts of growth. Scientists have shown renewed interest in exploring the development of various mature human capacities (here referred to as skills) and identifying factors that promote or cause development of these skills. Practitioners are beginning to think in terms of lags, deficits, or deviations in the normal developmental process. Classical diagnostic categories are being discarded for a more functional delineation of areas of adequate development and areas in which there is need for continued or redirected development.[1]

Treatment that emphasizes the nurturing of growth rests upon three major postulates: (1) Deviations in development can be altered.[2] (2) Subskills fundamental to mature adaptive skills must be acquired in a sequential manner.[3] (3) Mature adaptive skills can be acquired through participation in situations that simulate those interactions between individual and environment believed to be responsible for the sequential development of a given adaptive skill.[4]

© *AJOT XXIV, No. 4 May-June 1970. Reprinted with permission.*
This paper was presented at the annual conference of the AOTA in Dallas, TX, 1969.

It is out of this orientation, of treatment as recapitulation of ontogeny, that the concept of "developmental groups" has been formulated. It is presented principally as a heuristic device for discussing one facet of patient care.

Description of Developmental Groups

Developmental groups are clinical simulations of the various types of nonfamilial groups usually encountered in the normal developmental process.[5] These groups and their community-based counterparts are described as task-oriented and primary. Task-oriented refers to members' active engagement in the accomplishment of a definable project or task.[6] "A primary group is a face-to-face organization of individuals who cooperate for certain common ends, who share some common ideas and patterns of behavior, who have confidence in and some degree of affection for each other, and who are aware of their similarities of bonds of association."[7] The family (in its ideal form) is one example of a primary group. However, there are many nonfamilial groups that have the above listed characteristics. It is this type of group that is of concern in this paper.

Five types of developmental groups have been identified: parallel, project, egocentric-cooperative, cooperative and mature.[8] In a clinical setting, they would be described as follows:

A parallel group is made up of an aggregate of patients who are involved in individual tasks with minimal necessity for interaction. Group members may act as sources of stimulation for one another or tentatively test the effect of their behavior on others. However, task accomplishment does not require interaction. The therapist provides assistance with tasks and takes responsibility for meeting the social-emotional needs of each member.

In a project group, members are involved in common, short-term tasks that require some interaction, cooperation, and competition. The task is paramount. Mutual interaction outside the task is not expected. The therapist provides or assists the group in selecting tasks that require interaction of two or more persons for completion. He or she responds to the social-emotional needs of group members.

Egocentric-cooperative groups are characterized by group members selecting, implementing, and executing relatively long-term tasks through joint interaction. The task remains central but satisfaction of some social-emotional needs of fellow group members is encouraged. There is emphasis on the reciprocal satisfaction that can be gained by responding to others' needs. The therapist gives support and guidance relative to the task and continues to satisfy a considerable portion of each member's emotional needs.

In a cooperative group, members are encouraged to identify and gratify each other's social-emotional needs in conjuction with task accomplishment. This type of group often includes only members of the same sex. The therapist acts primarily in the role of an advisor and may not be present at all group meetings.

A mature group is heterogeneous in composition and characterized by members taking those task and social-emotional roles that are required for adequate group functioning. Maintenance of a proper balance between productivity and personal need satisfaction is stressed. The therapist interacts as a coequal group member.

Division of developmental groups into five types is arbitrary—an attempt to provide demarcation points. It is more accurate to perceive these groups as being on a continuum. Thus, in the clinical setting, a given group may be best described as standing somewhere between two adjacent types of developmental groups.

When used in the treatment process, developmental groups are seen as agents of planned change. It is postulated that change occurs through the individual experiencing the consequence of his behavior in the group setting.[9] Developmental groups are so structured that adaptive behavior leads to a positive reinforcing stimulus while maladaptive behavior does not. A positive reinforcing stimulus is an event that causes need reduction. The need may be outer-directed as in the need for companionship, or inner-directed as in the need to be competent.[10]

Treatment of Group Interaction Skill Deficiency

The concept of developmental groups was formulated originally to delineate and describe a method of treating deficiency in group interaction skill. It grew out of the attempt to apply recapitulation of ontogeny in the treatment of patients who were deficient in their ability to interact effectively in small groups. Although developmental groups may be utilized in other areas (which will be briefly discussed later) they are seen as particularly useful in treatment of inadequate development of group interaction skill.

Group interaction skill is here considered to be an adaptive skill. It is defined, in its mature form, as the ability to participate in a variety of groups in a manner that is satisfying for oneself and for one's fellow group members. It is postulated that this skill develops sequentially, each stage in its development being marked by acquisition of behavior that is required for adequate participation in the community-based counterpart of the five types of developmental groups. It is further postulated that group interaction skill is acquired through participation in these various types of groups in conjuction with the opportunity to experience the consequences of appropriate and inappropriate behavior.[11]

It is beyond the scope of this paper to give a detailed description of evaluative methods for group interaction skill. Ideally, the therapist and patient collaborate in identifying what stages of this skill the patient has successfully integrated. Pertinent information may be acquired by observation of the patient in a group situation and discussion with the patient about his participation in groups outside the clinical setting. Evaluation also involves identifying what behavior the patient needs to acquire for successful interaction in small groups and current behavior that is interfering with successful participation.

The therapist must determine when deficiency in group interaction skill will be dealt with in the treatment process. The criterion suggested for making this judgment is: treatment is initiated when the patient shows evidence of having acquired those abilities or skills that are normally learned prior to involvement in nonfamilial groups. The first step in treatment is engagement of the patient in that type of developmental group that is compatible or nearly compatible with his current capacity for meaningful group interaction.

Briefly, the treatment process consists of providing positive reinforcers for behaviors or approximation of behaviors that are necessary for successful participation in a given type of developmental group and withholding positive reinforcers for behaviors that are inconsistent with successful participation. These predetermined consequences are believed to be the central factor in bringing about change. The developmental group provides the structure; it sets and defines classes of behavior that are to be learned. Participation in a developmental group in and of itself is not conducive to planned behavioral change. Participation must be concurrent with deliberate and controlled reinforcement.

There are several methods that the therapist may use to increase the probability of the patient emitting desirable behavior so that they can be reinforced. The method or methods selected will be determined primarily by the other adaptive skills available to the patient and his fellow group members. The most primitive method is simply to wait until the patient exhibits an approximation of the behavior he needs to acquire. This behavior is differentially reinforced as it moves in the direction of becoming an affective behavior pattern. Other initiating methods are: (1) encouraging imitation of the therapist or other group members; (2) suggesting specific patterns of behavior to the patient; (3) identifying the patient's ineffectual responses and encouraging him to experiment with other forms of behavior; (4) group discussion regarding the behavior of self and others with mutual encouragement for engaging in appropriate and effective group behavior; and (5) experimentation with various behaviors through role-playing exercises.[12] Pragmatically, the therapist uses those initiating methods that appear to be successful.

An effort is made in all developmental groups to engage the patients in helping each other to acquire group interaction skill. Patients are encouraged to give and withhold reinforcers on the basis of the behavior exhibited by fellow group members. In order for patients to function as ancillary therapists, they must be able to comprehend what behavior is appropriate for a given type of developmental group and have sufficient self-control to give and withhold reinforcing stimuli. If it is deemed appropriate, the initial phase of treatment may be devoted to helping group members take on this ancillary therapist role.

Treatment continues to take place within the context of a specific type of developmental group until the patient has acquired the ability to function effectively in that group. He is then ready to begin learning the behavior that is necessary for competent functioning in the next, sequentially more advanced, developmental group. Depending upon the particular clinical situation and the extent to which the patient's fellow group members have progressed in an analogous manner, the patient is either placed in a new group or his original group as a whole is altered in the direction of the next type of developmental group. Treatment continues as previously outlined.

The treatment of deficiency in group interaction skill is terminated when any of the following criteria are met: (1) the patient has attained the ability to function in the type of group that is typical for his age. (2) He is able to participate in the kinds of groups that he is likely to encounter in his community environment (given its culture and the patient's preferred lifestyle). (3) The patient appears to be able to continue the development of group interaction skill outside the treatment situation.

Additional Comments

The concept of developmental groups was formulated in the attempt to apply recapitulation of ontogeny in the treatment of patients who were deficient in their ability to interact effectively in small groups. This concept may prove useful in three other areas. These areas are: (1) treatment of deficiency in other adaptive skills, (2) meeting mental health needs, and (3) describing the evolution of small groups.

Many of the subskills that are fundamental to the development of mature, adaptive skills are acquired through interaction in the familial group. These are usually the most basic or primitive subskills. However, more advanced subskills are often learned in the context of nonfamilial groups. The familial group may, indeed, continue to play a strongly supportive role, but interaction in nonfamilial groups is essential for adequate learning. (Treatment of those subskills that are usually developed within the family group is outside the scope of this paper.) In regard to those subskills that are partially or completely acquired through interaction in nonfamilial groups, it is suggested that they can be learned most easily through participation in a group that is structurally similar to the type of group in which the subskills are normally acquired. The concept of developmental groups could be used as a guide for selecting and forming appropriate groups. The difference between using developmental groups in the treatment of group interaction skill deficiency and deficiency in other adaptive skills is one of focus. The therapist would be primarily concerned with regulating reinforcement of behavior specific to the skill being learned as opposed to concentrating on helping the patient to learn how to function in the group. These two foci are not mutually exclusive, but it may be useful to deal with them as such to clarify treatment goals and methods.

That area of patient care here identified as meeting mental health needs refers to patient-therapist-nonhuman object interactions that are directed toward satisfying the normal human needs of the patient and maintaining his ability and desire to function.[13] The majority of mental health needs are most successfully met in a small group situation. However, needs cannot be satisfied unless there is synchronization of the individual's capacity to function in a particular group and the demands inherent in the structure of that group. In attempting to meet mental health needs, it is suggested that the therapist structure groups along a developmental continuum and that patients be encouraged to become involved in the type of group that is compatible with their group interaction skill. When a developmental group is oriented to satisfying mental health needs, the therapist is not concerned with bringing about a predetermined change in the patient's behavior. Therefore, the process of providing and withholding reinforcement is minimally important. The purpose of the group is to give pleasure, to have fun, to enjoy.

Preliminary, and somewhat superficial, observation indicates that the concept of developmental groups could be a useful tool in describing the evolution of task-oriented groups. This observation is not restricted to patient groups. As a task-oriented group moves toward becoming an effective working unit, there appear to be sequential patterns of interaction that are similar in many respects to the five types of developmental groups. Further study of this phenomenon may provide useful information for those persons who are concerned with facilitating the maturation and productivity of task-oriented groups.

The concept of developmental groups has been presented as a heuristic device. It is meant to stimulate interest and to encourage discovery. Its usefulness will be confirmed or refuted as we learn more about the human growth process, this entity that we call illness or dysfunction, and the effectiveness of treatment founded on the principles of recapitulation of ontogeny.

References

1. A. Jean Ayres, "Perceptual Motor Dysfunction in Children," paper presented at the Ohio Occupational Therapy Association Conference, 1964; John Flavell, *The Developmental Psychology of Jean Piaget* (New York: D. Van Nostrand Company, 1963); Anne Mosey, *Occupational Therapy: Theory and Practice* (printed through support of R.S.A. Training Grant No. 543-T-65 by Pothier Brothers, Medford, MA 1968); Maya Pines, "Why Some 3-Year Olds Get A's-and Some Get C's", *The New York Times Magazine*, July 6, 1969; Kenneth Overly, "Developmental Theory and Occupational Therapy-Considerations for Research," paper presented at the American Occupational Therapy Association Convention, Portland, Oregon, 1968; Marguerite Sechehaye, *A New Psychotherapy in Schizophrenia* (New York: Grune and Stratton, 1965).
2. Overly, "Developmental Theory and Occupational Therapy...."
3. Flavell, *The Developmental Psychology of Jean Piaget.*
4. Ayres, *Perceptual Motor Dysfunction in Children;* Mosey, *Occupational Therapy....*
5. Mosey, *Occupational Therapy....*
6. Gail Fidler, "The Task-Oriented Group as a Context for Treatment", *American Journal of Occupational Therapy*, 23, (1969).
7. H. English and A. English, *A Comprehensive Dictionary of Psychological and Psychoanalytic Terms* (New York: David McKay Co., 1958).
8. Erik Erikson, *Childhood and Society* (New York: W.W. Norton and Co., 1950); Anna Freud, *Normality and Pathology in Childhood* (New York: International Universities Press, 1965); T. Parsons and R. Bales, *Family, Socialization and the Interaction Process* (Glencoe, IL: The Free Press, 1955); J. Pearce and S. Newton, *The*

Conditions of Human Growth (New York: Citadel Press, 1963).

9. C. Ferster and M. Perrott, *Behavior Principles* (New York: Appleton-Century-Crofts, 1961); Gregory Kimble, *Hilgard and Margis' Conditioning and Learning* (New York: Appleton-Century-Crofts, 1961); B.F. Skinner, *Science and Human Behavior* (New York: The Macmillan Co., 1953); A. Smith and V. Tempone, "Psychiatric Occupational Therapy Within a Learning Theory Context", *American Journal of Occupational Therapy* (September-October 1968); Kenneth Spence, *Behavior Theory and Conditioning* (New Haven, CT: Yale University Press, 1956).

10. Spence, *Behavior Theory and Conditioning*

11. Parsons and Bales, *Family, Socialization, and the Interaction Process*; George Mead, *Mind, Self and Society* (Chicago, IL: University of Chicago Press, 1934); Theodore Mills, *The Sociology of Small Groups* (Englewood Cliffs, NJ: Prentice-Hall, 1963).

12. Fidler, "The Task-Oriented Group...."

13. G. Fidler and J. Fidler, *Occupational Therapy: A Communication Process in Psychiatry* (New York: The Macmillan Company, 1963).

Appendix
C

Summary of Mosey's Adaptive Skills

Sensory Integration Skill: The ability to receive, select, combine, and coordinate vestibular, proprioceptive, and tactile information for functional use.
1. The ability to integrate the tactile subsystems (birth-3 months).
2. The ability to integrate primitive postural reflexes (3-9 months).
3. Maturation of mature righting and equilibrium reactions (9-12 months).
4. The ability to integrate the two sides of the body, to be aware of body parts and their relationship, and to plan gross motor movements (1-2 yr).
5. The ability to plan fine motor movements (2-3 yr).

Cognitive Skill: The ability to perceive, represent, and organize sensory information for the purpose of thinking and problem-solving.
1. The ability to use inherent behavioral patterns for environmental interaction (birth-1 month).
2. The ability to interrelate visual, manual, auditory, and oral responses (1-4 months).
3. The ability to attend to the environmental consequence of actions with interest, to represent objects in an exoceptual manner, to experience objects, to act on the bases of egocentric causality, and to seriate events in which the self is involved (4-9 months).
4. The ability to establish a goal and intentionally carry out means, to recognize the independent existence of objects, to interpret signs, to imitate new behavior to apprehend the influence of space, and to perceive other objects as partially causal (9-12 months).
5. The ability to use trial-and-error problem-solving, to use tools, to perceive variability in spacial positions, to seriate events in which the self is not involved, and to perceive the causality of other objects (12-18 months).
6. The ability to represent objects in an image manner, to make believe, to infer a cause given its effect, to act on the bases of combined spatial relations, to attribute omnipotence to others, and to perceive objects as permanent in time and place (18 months-2 yr).

7. The ability to represent objects in an endoceptual manner, to differentiate between thought and action, and to recognize the need for causal sources (2-5 yr).
8. The ability to represent objects in a denotative manner, to perceive the viewpoint of others, and to decenter (6-7 yr).
9. The ability to represent objects in a connotative manner, to use formal logic, and to work in the realm of the hypothetical (11-13 yr).

Dyadic Interaction Skill: The ability to participate in a variety of dyadic relationships.
1. The ability to enter into trusting familial relationships (8-10 months).
2. The ability to enter into association relationships (3-5 yr).
3. The ability to interact in an authority relationship (5-7 yr).
4. The ability to interact in a chum relationship (10-14 yr).
5. The ability to enter into a peer, authority relationship (15-17 yr).
6. The ability to enter into an intimate relationship (18-25 yr).
7. The ability to engage in a nurturing relationship (20-30 yr).

Group Interaction Skill: The ability to engage in a variety of primary groups.
1. The ability to participate in a parallel group (18 months-2 yr).
2. The ability to participate in a project group (2-4 yr).
3. The ability to participate in an egocentric group (9-12 yr).
4. The ability to participate in a cooperative group (9-12 yr).
5. The ability to participate in a mature group (15-18 yr).

Self-Identity Skill: The ability to perceive the self as a relatively autonomous, holistic, and acceptable person who has permanence and continuity over time.
1. The ability to perceive the self as a worthy person (9-12 months).
2. The ability to perceive the assets and limitations of the self (11-15 yr).
3. The ability to perceive the self as self-directed (20-25 yr)
4. The ability to perceive the self as a productive, contributing member of a social system (30-35 yr).
5. The ability to perceive the self as having an autonomous identity (35-50 yr).
6. The ability to perceive the aging process of oneself and ultimate death as part of the life cycle (45-60 yr).

Sexual Identity Skill: The ability to perceive one's sexual nature as good and to participate in a relatively long-term sexual relationship that is oriented to the mutual satisfaction of sexual needs.
1. The ability to accept and act on the basis of one's pregenital sexual nature (4-5 yr).
2. The ability to accept sexual maturation as a positive growth experience (12-16 yr).
3. The ability to give and receive sexual gratification (18-25 yr).
4. The ability to enter into a sustained sexual relationship characterized by the mutual satisfaction of sexual needs (20-30 yr).
5. The ability to accept the sex-related physiological changes that occur as a natural part of the aging process (40-60 yr).

From Mosey A. *Psychosocial Components of Occupational Therapy*, Raven Press, New York, 1986. Reprinted with permission.

Appendix

D

Uniform Terminology For Reporting Occupational Therapy Services, Third Edition

Used by permission of The American Occupational Therapy Association, Inc., Rockville, Maryland

"Occupational Therapy" is the use of purposeful activity or interventions to promote health and achieve functional outcomes. "Achieving functional outcomes" means to develop, improve, or restore the highest possible level of independence of any individual who is limited by a physical injury or illness, a dysfunctional condition, a cognitive impairment, a psychosocial dysfunction, a mental illness, a developmental or learning disability, or an adverse environmental condition. Assessment means the use of skilled observation or evaluation by the administration and interpretation of standardized or nonstandardized tests and measurements to identify areas for occupational therapy services.

Occupational therapy services include, but are not limited to:

1. the assessment, treatment, and education of or consultation with the individual, family, or other persons;
2. interventions directed toward developing, improving, or restoring daily living skills, work readiness or work performance, play skills or leisure capacities, or enhancing educational performances skills; or
3. providing for the development, improvement, or restoration of sensorimotor, oral-motor, perceptual or neuromuscular functioning; or emotional, motivational, cognitive, or psychosocial components of performance.

These services may require assessment of the need for and use of interventions such as the design, development, adaptation, application, or training in the use of assistive technology devices; the design, fabrication, or application of rehabilitative technology such as selected orthotic devices; training in the use of assistive technology, orthotic or prosthetic devices; the application of physical agent modalities as an adjunct to or in preparation for purposeful activity; the use of ergonomic principles; the adaptation of environments and processes to enhance functional performance; or the promotion of health and wellness (AOTA, 1993, p. 1117).

I. Performance Areas

Throughout this document, activities have been described as if individuals performed the tasks themselves. Occupational therapy also recognizes that individuals arrange for tasks to be done through others. The profession views independence as the ability to self-determine activity performance, regardless of who actually performs the activity.

A. *Activities of Daily Living*—Self-maintenance tasks.

1. *Grooming*—Obtaining and using supplies; removing body hair (use of razors, tweezers, lotions, etc.); applying and removing cosmetics; washing, drying, combing, styling, and brushing hair; caring for nails (hands and feet), caring for skin, ears, and eyes; and applying deodorant.

2. *Oral Hygiene*—Obtaining and using supplies; cleaning mouth; brushing and flossing teeth; or removing, cleaning, and reinserting dental orthotics and prosthetics.

3. *Bathing/Showering*—Obtaining and using supplies; soaping, rinsing, and drying all body parts; maintaining bathing position; transferring to and from bathing positions.

4. *Toilet Hygiene*—Obtaining and using supplies; clothing management; maintaining toileting position; transferring to and from toileting position; cleaning body; and caring for menstrual and continence needs (including catheters, colostomies, and suppository management).

5. *Personal Device Care*—Cleaning and maintaining personal care items, such as hearing aids, contact lenses, glasses, orthotics, prosthetics, adaptive equipment, and contraceptive and sexual devices.

6. *Dressing*—Selecting clothing and accessories appropriate for the time of day, weather, and occasion; obtaining clothing from storage area; dressing and undressing in a sequential fashion; fastening and adjusting clothing and shoes; and applying and removing personal devices, prostheses, or orthoses.

7. *Feeding and Eating*—Setting up food; selecting and using appropriate utensils and tableware; bringing food or drink to mouth; sucking, masticating, coughing, and swallowing; and management of alternative methods or nourishment.

8. *Medication Routine*—Obtaining medication, opening and closing containers, following prescribed schedules, taking correct quantities, reporting problems and adverse effects, and administering correct quantities using prescribed methods.

9. *Health Maintenance*—Developing and maintaining routines for illness prevention and wellness promotion, such as physical fitness, nutrition, and decreasing health risk behaviors.

10. *Socialization*—Accessing opportunities and interacting with other people in appropriate contextual and cultural ways to meet emotional and physical needs.

11. *Functional Communication*—Using equipment or systems to send and receive information, such as writing equipment, telephones, typewriters, communication boards, call lights, emergency systems, Braille writers, telecommunication devices for the deaf, and augmentative communication systems.

12. *Functional Mobility*—Moving from one position or place to another, such as in-bed mobility, wheelchair mobility, transfers (wheelchair, bed, car, tub/shower, toilet, chair, floor); performing functional ambulation and transporting objects.

13. *Community Mobility*—Moving self in the community and using public or private transportation, such as driving, or accessing buses, taxi cabs, or other public transportation systems.

14. *Emergency Response*—Recognizing sudden, unexpected hazardous situations, and initiating action to reduce the threat to health and safety.

15. *Sexual Expression*—Engaging in desired sexual activities.

B. *Work and Productive Activities*—Purposeful activities for self-development, social contribution, and livelihood.

1. *Home Management*—Obtaining and maintaining personal and household possessions and environment.

    a. *Clothing Care*—Obtaining and using supplies; sorting, laundering (hand, machine, and dry clean); folding; ironing; storing; and mending.

    b. *Cleaning*—Obtaining and using supplies; picking up; putting away; vacuuming; sweeping and mopping floors; dusting; polishing; scrubbing; washing windows; cleaning mirrors; making beds; and removing trash and recyclables.

    c. *Meal Preparation and Cleanup*—Planning nutritious meals; preparing and serving food; opening and closing containers, cabinets, and drawers; using kitchen utensils and appliances; cleaning up and storing food safely.

    d. *Shopping*—Preparing shopping lists (grocery and other); selecting and purchasing items; selecting method of payment; and completing money transactions.

    e. *Money Management*—Budgeting, paying bills, and using bank systems.

    f. *Household Maintenance*—Maintaining home, yard, garden appliances, vehicles, and household items.

    g. *Safety Procedures*—Knowing and performing preventive and emergency procedures to maintain a safe environment and prevent injuries.

2. *Care of Others*—Providing for children, spouse, parents, pets or others, such as the physical care, nurturing, communicating, and using age-appropriate activities.

3. *Educational Activities*—Participating in a learning environment through school, community, or work-sponsored activities, such as exploring educational interests, attending to instruction, managing assignments, and contributing to group experiences.

4. *Vocational Activities*—Participating in work-related activities.

    a. *Vocational Exploration*—Determining aptitudes, developing interests and skills, and selecting appropriate vocational pursuits.

    b. *Job Acquisition*—Identifying and selecting work opportunities, and completing application and interview processes.

    c. *Work or Job Performance*—Performing job tasks in a timely and effective manner; incorporating necessary work behaviors.

    d. *Retirement Planning*—Determining aptitudes, developing interests and skills, and identifying appropriate avocational pursuits.

    e. *Volunteer Participation*—Performing unpaid activities for the benefit of selected individuals, groups, or causes.

C. *Play or Leisure Activities*—Intrinsically motivating activities for amusement, relaxation, spontaneous enjoyment, or self-expression.

1. *Play or Leisure Exploration*—Identifying interests, skills, opportunities, and appropriate play or leisure activities.

2. *Play or Leisure Performance*—Planning and participating in play or leisure activities; maintaining a balance of play or leisure activities with work and productive activities, and activities of daily living; obtaining, utilizing, and maintaining equipment and supplies.

II. Performance Components

A. *Sensorimotor Component*—The ability to receive input, process information, and produce output.

1. *Sensory*

    a. *Sensory Awareness*—Receiving and differentiating sensory stimuli.

    b. *Sensory Processing*—Interpreting sensory stimuli.

        (1) *Tactile*—Interpreting light touch, pressure, temperature, pain, and vibration through skin contact/receptors.

        (2) *Proprioceptive*—Interpreting stimuli originating in muscles, joints, and other internal tissues to give information about the position of one body part in relation to another.

        (3) *Vestibular*—Interpreting stimuli from the inner ear receptors regarding head position and movement.

        (4) *Visual*—Interpreting stimuli through the eyes, including peripheral vision and acuity, awareness of color and pattern.

(5) *Auditory*—Interpreting and localizing sounds, and discriminating background sounds.

(6) *Gustatory*—Interpreting tastes.

(7) *Olfactory*—Interpreting odors.

c. *Perceptual Processing*—Organizing sensory input into meaningful patterns.

(1) *Stereognosis*—Identifying objects through proprioception, cognition, and the sense of touch.

(2) *Kinesthesia*—Identifying the excursion and direction of joint movement.

(3) *Pain Response*—Interpreting noxious stimuli.

(4) *Body Scheme*—Acquiring an internal awareness of the body and the relationship of body parts to each other.

(5) *Right-Left Discrimination*—Differentiating one side of the body from the other.

(6) *Form Constancy*—Recognizing forms and objects as the same in various environments, positions, and sizes.

(7) *Position in Space*—Determining the spatial relationship of figures and objects to self or other forms and objects.

(8) *Visual-Closure*—Identifying forms or objects from incomplete presentations.

(9) *Figure Ground*—Differentiating between foreground and background forms and objects.

(10) *Depth Perception*—Determining the relative distance between objects, figures, or landmarks and the observer, and changes in planes of surfaces.

(11) *Spatial Relations*—Determining the position of objects relative to each other.

(12) *Topographical Orientation*—Determining the location of objects and settings and the route to the location.

2. *Neuromusculoskeletal*

a. *Reflex*—Eliciting an involuntary muscle response by sensory input.

b. *Range of Motion*—Moving body parts through an arc.

c. *Muscle Tone*—Demonstrating a degree of tension or resistance in a muscle at rest and in response to stretch.

d. *Strength*—Demonstrating a degree of muscle power when movement is resisted, as with objects or gravity.

e. *Endurance*—Sustaining cardiac, pulmonary, and musculoskeletal exertion over time.

f. *Postural Control*—Using righting and equilibrium adjustments to maintain balance during functional movements.

g. *Postural Alignment*—Maintaining biomechanical integrity among body parts.

h. *Soft Tissue Integrity*—Maintaining anatomical and physiological condition of interstitial tissue and skin.

3. *Motor*

a. *Gross Coordination*—Using large muscle groups for controlled, goal-directed movements.

b. *Crossing the Midline*—Moving limbs and eyes across the midsagittal plane of the body.

c. *Laterality*—Using a preferred unilateral body part for activities requiring a high level of skill.

d. *Bilateral Integration*—Coordinating both body sides during activity.

e. *Motor Control*—Using the body in functional and versatile movement patterns.

f. *Praxis*—Conceiving and planning a new motor act in response to an environmental demand.

g. *Fine Coordination/Dexterity*—Using small muscle groups for controlled movements, particularly in object manipulation.

h. *Visual-Motor Integration*—Coordinating the interaction of information from the eyes with body movement during activity.

i. *Oral-Motor Control*—Coordinating oropharyngeal musculature for controlled movements.

B. *Cognitive Integration and Cognitive Components*

1. *Level of Arousal*—Demonstrating alertness and responsiveness to environmental stimuli.

2. *Orientation*—Identifying person, place, time, and situation.

3. *Recognition*—Identifying familiar faces, objects, and other previously presented materials.
4. *Attention Span*—Focusing on a task over time.
5. *Initiation of Activity*—Starting a physical or mental activity.
6. *Termination of Activity*—Stopping an activity at an appropriate time.
7. *Memory*—Recalling information after brief or long periods of time.
8. *Sequencing*—Placing information, concepts, and actions in order.
9. *Categorization*—Identifying similarities of and differences among pieces of environmental information.
10. *Concept Formation*—Organizing a variety of information to form thoughts and ideas.
11. *Spatial Operations*—Mentally manipulating the position of objects in various relationships.
12. *Problem Solving*—Recognizing a problem, defining a problem, identifying alternative plans, selecting a plan, organizing steps in a plan, implementing a plan, and evaluating the outcome.
13. *Learning*—Acquiring new concepts and behaviors.
14. *Generalization*—Applying previously learned concepts and behaviors to a variety of new situations.

C. *Psychosocial Skills and Psychological Components*—The ability to interact in society and to process emotions.
   1. *Psychological*
      a. *Values*—Identifying ideas or beliefs that are important to self and others.
      b. *Interests*—Identifying mental or physical activities that create pleasure and maintain attention.
      c. *Self-Concept*—Developing the value of the physical, emotional, and sexual self.
   2. *Social*
      a. *Role Performance*—Identifying, maintaining, and balancing functions one assumes or acquires in society (e.g., worker, student, parent, friend, religious participant).
      b. *Social Conduct*—Interacting using manners, personal space, eye contact, gestures, active listening, and self-expression appropriate to one's environment.
      c. *Interpersonal Skills*—Using verbal and nonverbal communication to interact in a variety of settings.
      d. *Self-Expression*—Using a variety of styles and skills to express thoughts, feelings, and needs.
   3. *Self-Management*
      a. *Coping Skills*—Identifying and managing stress and related reactors.
      b. *Time Management*—Planning and participating in a balance of self-care, work, leisure, and rest activities to promote satisfaction and health.
      c. *Self-Control*—Modifying one's own behavior in response to environmental needs, demands, constraints, personal aspirations, and feedback from others.

III. **Performance Contexts**

Assessment of function in performance areas is greatly influenced by the contexts in which the individual must perform. Occupational therapy practitioners consider performance contexts when determining feasibility and appropriateness of interventions. Occupational therapy practitioners may choose interventions based on an understanding of contexts, or may choose interventions directly aimed at altering the contexts to improve performance.

A. *Temporal Aspects*
   1. *Chronological*—Individual's age.
   2. *Developmental*—Stage or phase of maturation.
   3. *Life Cycle*—Place in important life phases, such as career cycle, parenting cycle, or educational process.
   4. *Disability Status*—Place in continuum of disability, such as acuteness of injury, chronicity of disability, or terminal nature of illness.

B. *Environment*

1. *Physical*—Nonhuman aspects of contexts. Includes the accessibility to and performance within environments having natural terrain, plants, animals, buildings, furniture, objects, tools, or devices.
2. *Social*—Availability and expectations of significant individuals, such as spouse, friends, and caregivers. Also includes larger social groups which are influential in establishing norms, role expectations, and social routines.
3. *Cultural*—Customs, beliefs, activity patterns, behavior standards, and expectations accepted by the society of which the individual is a member. Includes political aspects, such as laws that affect access to resources and affirm personal rights. Also includes opportunities for education, employment, and economic support.

References

American Occupational Therapy Association. (1979). *Occupational therapy output reporting system and uniform terminology for reporting occupational therapy services.* Rockville, MD: Author.

American Occupational Therapy Association. (1989). Uniform terminology for occupational therapy—Second edition. *American Journal of Occupational Therapy, 43,* 808-815.

American Occupational Therapy Association. (1993). Definition of occupational therapy practice for state regulation (Policy 5.3.1). *American Journal of Occupational Therapy, 47,* 1117-1121.

Authors:

The Terminology Task Force:
  Winifred Dunn, PhD, OTR, FAOTA—Chairperson
  Mary Foto, OTR, FAOTA
  Jim Hinojosa, PhD, OTR, FAOTA
  Barbara Schell, PhD, OTR/L, FAOTA
  Linda Kohlman Thomson, MOT, OTR, OT(C), FAOTA
  Sarah D. Hertfelder, MEd, MOT, OTR/L—Staff Liaison

for The Commission on Practice
Jim Hinojosa, PhD, OTR, FAOTA—Chairperson
Adopted by the Representative Assembly 7/94

> **NOTE:** This document replaces the following documents, all of which were rescinded by the 1994 Representative Assembly:

Occupational Therapy Product Output Reporting System (1979)
Uniform Terminology for Reporting Occupational Therapy Services—First Edition (1979)
Uniform Occupational Therapy Evaluation Checklist (1981)
Uniform Terminology for Occupational Therapy—Second Edition (1989)

Appendix
E

Comparison of Group Leadership Guidelines in Seven Frames of Reference

By Marilyn B. Cole, MS, OTR/L

EXISTENTIAL/HUMANISTIC

STRUCTURE	loosely structured, discussion oriented
TIME	one hour or longer
GOALS	self understanding insight, self- actualization
LEADERSHIP	facilitator/advisor
ACTIVITY GUIDELINES	involve self-disclosure and interaction
1. Introduction	members acknowledged introduce ground rules
2. Activity	explore meaning of life and personal values
3. Sharing	feedback and mutual acceptance and empathy
4. Processing	feelings explored thoroughly
5. Generalizing	principles learned are elicited from members
6. Application	members speak about how they will personally apply principles
7. Summary	members contribute to summary

COGNITIVE

STRUCTURE	highly structured with specific short term goals based on cognitive level
TIME	30-60 minutes based on member attention span
GOALS	specific, observable, measurable, focus on learning skills
LEADERSHIP	director/educator, therapist instructs and assists throughout activity
ACTIVITY GUIDELINES	should focus on alteration of thought process, attention, perception, problem-solving, motor action and conscious awareness
1. Introduction	no warm-up, focus on elaboration of goals and purpose
2. Activity	task performance, goals emphasized; activity takes most of session
3. Sharing	minimal
4. Processing	impact of feeling on thinking or learning may be explored but not emphasized
5. Generalizing	inductive reasoning is encouraged in higher level groups only
6. Application	members encouraged to practice applying new skills in specific situations
7. Summary	purpose is to reinforce learning

PSYCHOANALYTIC

STRUCTURE	loosely structured, task oriented
TIME	one hour
GOALS	ego skill development and strengthening
LEADERSHIP	facilitator
ACTIVITY GUIDELINES	members project self through activities
1. Introduction	purpose explained
2. Activity	phase 1: planning a task phase 2: doing a task
3. Sharing	all members choose and take part in task
4. Processing	phase 3: evaluating, feelings elicited and problems explored
5. Generalizing	done at end of each session;
6. Application	feedback is given to members to strengthen functions of the ego
7. Summary	therapist leads discussion

DEVELOPMENTAL

STRUCTURE	homogeneous groups work on specific age-appropriate skills in growth facilitating environment
TIME	30-90 minutes, increases with maturity
GOALS	master skills needed to progress to next higher level of development
LEADERSHIP	director, therapist sets up environment and plans activity
ACTIVITY GUIDELINES	based on life tasks appropriate to age and stage of development in social, psychological, intellectual or moral developmental theory
1. Introduction	names, warm-up, structure and purpose explained
2. Activity	graded to follow developmental guidelines matching stages of members
3. Sharing	self-expression and feedback are encouraged
4. Processing	feelings about both past and present experience are shared
5. Generalizing	therapist guides discussion of general principles along developmental lines
6. Application	each member applies new skills to his/her own life
7. Summary	stress application of learning for growth

NEURODEVELOPMENTAL

STRUCTURE	highly structured sequence of sensory motor activities
TIME	30-60 minutes
GOALS	stimulate development of central nervous system, adaptive functioning and a sense of calm alertness
LEADERSHIP	directive, role-modeling and imitation used to guide
ACTIVITY GUIDELINES	movement oriented, according to specific theorist
1. Introduction	acknowledge, approach movement cautiously, use introduction to gauge tolerance
2. Activity	focus on movement and sensory stimulation
3. Sharing	non-verbal
4. Processing	verbalize feelings about activity
5. Generalizing	done by therapist in summary
6. Application	spontaneous
7. Summary	summarize learning and expected outcome

ACQUISITIONAL

STRUCTURE	highly structured, minimal interaction, members reinforce each other
TIME	30-60 minutes
GOALS	specific, observable and measurable, patient has input, improve functional performance
LEADERSHIP	directive, therapist instructs, assists, and provides cuing
ACTIVITY GUIDELINES	strength, endurance, attention, perception, communication, cognition and skills of daily living
1. Introduction	no warm-up, communicate specific expectations, and purpose geared to member understanding
2. Activity	one or several tasks focusing on specific skills in a specific environment
3. Sharing	materials not shared; results shared to learn from each other
4. Processing	discuss how feelings impact learning
5. Generalizing	therapist assists members in generalizing skills from optimal learning environment to discharge environment
6. Application	members discuss how they will apply learning, also communicated to caretakers
7. Summary	reinforces learning

MODEL OF HUMAN OCCUPATION

STRUCTURE	not identified
TIME	wide range, 1 hour to several days
GOALS	restore order to daily occupation
LEADERSHIP	facilitator/advisor patient is given choices
ACTIVITY GUIDELINES	normal daily activities: work, play, self-care at levels of exploration, competence and achievement
1. Introduction	names, warm-up optional, purpose discussed thoroughly with patient input
2. Activity	work on tasks/ skills needed to perform life roles of members
3. Sharing	not necessary
4. Processing	not necessary
5. Generalizing	meaning of activity with regard to system efficiency and meaningful occupational performance is discussed
6. Application	individual performance is discussed and compared with demands of intended environment
7. Summary	review goals and acknowledge individual achievement

Index

of reference, 110-111
complaining behavior, group dynamics, 51
concepts, reformulation of, for treatment guidelines, 62
conceptual framework
combination with postulate, 62
selection of, 61-62
concreteness, existential/humanistic therapeutic frame of reference, 74-75
confrontation, existential/humanistic therapeutic frame of reference, 82-83
consensual validation, psychoanalytic therapeutic frame of reference, 103
content-process, in group dynamics, reaction worksheet, 31
contract, student, for group membership, 268
control stage, group dynamics, 33-34
cooperative groups, psychoanalytic therapeutic frame of reference, 115
cost, group treatment protocol writing, 239

death, coming to terms with, developmental therapeutic frame of reference, 157-158
defense mechanisms, psychoanalytic therapeutic frame of reference, 108-110
description, group treatment protocol writing, 239
destruction/creation polarity, developmental therapeutic frame of reference, 155
developmental group, use of, 281-286
developmental therapeutic frame of reference
activity, 162-169
application, 169
basic assumptions, 150-159
change, 160-161
death, coming to terms with, 157-158
destruction/creation polarity, 155
dysfunction, 160
early adult transition, 152-154
Erikson, E., 150-151
function, 160
generalizing, 169
Gilligan, C., 159
group leadership, 167-169
group treatment in, 161-167
Jung, C., 150-151
late adult transition, 156-158
leader, role of, 162
Levinson, D., 151-158
life structure modification, 154-155
marriage, 153-154
masculine/feminine polarity, 155-156
mentor relationship, 153

mid-life individuation, 155
mid-life transition, 154-155
motivation, 160-161
occupation selection, 153
physical decline, 156-157
processing, 169
productive role, loss of, 157
reappraisal of past, 154
sharing, 169
Wilcox, M., 158-159
young/old polarity, 155
directive leadership, activity groups, 17
dysfunction
acquisitional frame of reference, 213-214
developmental therapeutic frame of reference, 160
existential/humanistic therapeutic frame of reference, 69
model of human occupation therapeutic frame of reference, 197
neurodevelopmental therapeutic frame of reference, 182-183
psychoanalytic therapeutic frame of reference, 111

early adult transition, developmental therapeutic frame of reference, 152-154
ego
psychoanalytic therapeutic frame of reference, 100
psychology, assumptions of, psychoanalytic therapeutic frame of reference, 103-111
egocentric-cooperative groups, psychoanalytic therapeutic frame of reference, 115
Ellis, A., cognitive therapeutic frame of reference, 131-132
empathy
advanced accurate, existential/humanistic therapeutic frame of reference, 80-81
primary accurate, existential/humanistic therapeutic frame of reference, 76-78
endurance, acquisitional frame of reference, 208-209
environmental interaction, model of human occupation therapeutic frame of reference, 195-196
Erikson, E., developmental therapeutic frame of reference, 150-151
evaluation worksheet, group treatment plan sample, 267
exercise groups, neurodevelopmental therapeutic frame of reference, 188-189
existential concepts, existential/humanistic ther-